The Research-Backed Anti-Inflammatory Diet Cookbook For Beginners

365 Days of No-Stress Recipes to Enhanced Immune System, Relief Pain, Reduce Inflammation and Promotes Overall Well-being | 28-Day Meal Plan & Full Color Pictures Included

TIMOTHY A. GWIN

Copyright Page

TABLE OF CONTENTS

INTRODUCTION

Inflammation – it's a term we often hear in discussions about health and wellness, but what exactly does it mean? And why is it important to consider when it comes to our diet and overall well-being? The Introduction section of "The Research-Backed Anti-Inflammatory Diet Cookbook For Beginners" sets the stage by providing a comprehensive overview of inflammation and its impact on health, while also delving into the benefits of adopting an anti-inflammatory diet.

UNDERSTANDING INFLAMMATION AND ITS IMPACT ON HEALTH

To kick things off, this subsection delves deep into the concept of inflammation, breaking down the complex biological processes that occur within the body in response to various triggers such as injury, infection, or chronic stress. Readers will gain a clear understanding of how inflammation manifests, from the classic signs of redness, swelling, and pain to the less obvious internal inflammation that can silently wreak havoc on our health.

Moreover, the section explores the distinction between acute and chronic inflammation, emphasizing the latter's role in the development and progression of numerous chronic diseases, including heart disease, diabetes, arthritis, and even certain cancers. By providing this foundational knowledge, readers are empowered to recognize the importance of managing inflammation through lifestyle choices, particularly dietary interventions.

BENEFITS OF ANTI-INFLAMMATORY DIET

- **Reduction of Chronic Inflammation:** Chronic inflammation is linked to the development and progression of various diseases, including heart disease, diabetes, cancer, and autoimmune disorders. An anti-inflammatory diet can help to reduce systemic inflammation throughout the body, thereby lowering the risk of these chronic conditions.

- **Improved Heart Health:** Many of the foods emphasized in an anti-inflammatory diet, such as fruits, vegetables, whole grains, nuts, and fatty fish, are also heart-healthy. By reducing inflammation and promoting healthy cholesterol levels, blood pressure, and blood sugar regulation, an anti-inflammatory diet can significantly improve cardiovascular health and reduce the risk of heart disease and stroke.

- **Better Management of Autoimmune Conditions:** Autoimmune diseases occur when the immune system mistakenly attacks healthy tissues in the body. Since inflammation is a key driver of autoimmune disorders, an anti-inflammatory diet can help to mitigate symptoms and improve quality of life for individuals living with conditions such as rheumatoid arthritis, lupus, and inflammatory bowel disease.

- **Enhanced Joint Health:** Inflammatory arthritis conditions like rheumatoid arthritis and psoriatic arthritis can cause pain, stiffness, and swelling in the joints.

- By reducing inflammation in the body, an anti-inflammatory diet may help to alleviate symptoms and improve joint function, allowing individuals to better manage their condition and maintain mobility.
- **Support for Brain Health:** Chronic inflammation has been implicated in cognitive decline and neurodegenerative diseases such as Alzheimer's and Parkinson's. Antioxidant-rich foods and omega-3 fatty acids found in abundance in an anti-inflammatory diet have been shown to support brain health, protect against oxidative stress, and potentially reduce the risk of age-related cognitive decline.
- **Weight Management:** Obesity is associated with low-grade chronic inflammation, which can further contribute to metabolic dysfunction and increase the risk of chronic diseases like type 2 diabetes and cardiovascular disease. By promoting weight loss and reducing inflammation, an anti-inflammatory diet can help individuals achieve and maintain a healthy weight, improving overall metabolic health and reducing disease risk.
- **Gut Health:** The gut microbiome plays a crucial role in regulating inflammation and immune function throughout the body. Certain dietary factors, such as fiber-rich fruits and vegetables and fermented foods like yogurt and kefir, can promote a healthy balance of gut bacteria and reduce gut inflammation, supporting digestive health and overall well-being.
- **Improved Skin Health:** Inflammatory skin conditions like acne, eczema, and psoriasis can be exacerbated by dietary factors that promote inflammation. By focusing on whole, nutrient-dense foods and avoiding pro-inflammatory triggers like processed sugars and refined carbohydrates, an anti-inflammatory diet may help to improve skin health and reduce the severity of these conditions.

HOW TO USE THIS COOKBOOK

This cookbook is designed to be a practical guide to help you implement the principles of the Anti-Inflammatory Diet into your daily life. Here's how to make the most of it:

- **Understand the Basics:** Begin by familiarizing yourself with the core principles of the Anti-Inflammatory Diet. Read through the introductory sections to understand the science behind the diet and the recommended foods and practices.
- **Meal Planning:** Use the cookbook to plan your meals. The recipes are categorized by meal type—breakfast, lunch, dinner, and snacks—to make it easy to find what you need. Planning your meals ahead of time can help ensure you have the necessary ingredients and can adhere to the diet more easily.
- **Grocery Shopping:** Take advantage of the shopping lists provided in the cookbook. These lists are tailored to the recipes and ensure you have all the ingredients needed to prepare anti-inflammatory, nutrient-dense meals.
- **Cooking Techniques:** Follow the step-by-step instructions in each recipe. The cookbook includes tips on cooking techniques and modifications to suit different dietary needs and preferences.
- **Incorporate Intermittent Fasting:** The cookbook provides guidance on how to time your meals and snacks to align with your fasting periods.
- **Mindful Eating:** Practice mindful eating by savoring each meal and paying attention to hunger and satiety cues. The cookbook encourages you to enjoy the process of cooking and eating, making it a pleasurable and rewarding part of your day.
- **Track Your Progress:** Keep a journal of your meals, symptoms, and any changes you notice in your health. Tracking your progress can help you identify patterns and make adjustments as needed.

BASICS OF ANTI-INFLAMMATORY EATING

Inflammation is a natural process that helps your body heal and defend itself from harm. However, when inflammation becomes chronic, it can contribute to various health problems, including heart disease, diabetes, arthritis, and even certain cancers. The goal of an anti-inflammatory diet is to reduce chronic inflammation, promote overall health, and help prevent or manage these conditions.

PRINCIPLES OF ANTI-INFLAMMATORY EATING

An anti-inflammatory diet focuses on whole, nutrient-dense foods that can help reduce inflammation. Key principles include:

- **Emphasizing Fruits and Vegetables:** These are rich in antioxidants, vitamins, and minerals. Aim for a colorful variety to ensure a wide range of nutrients.
- **Choosing Healthy Fats:** Incorporate sources of omega-3 fatty acids, such as fatty fish (salmon, mackerel), flaxseeds, and walnuts. Use olive oil for cooking and dressings.
- **Opting for Whole Grains:** Whole grains like quinoa, brown rice, and oats provide fiber and nutrients. Avoid refined grains and sugars.
- **Including Lean Proteins:** Focus on plant-based proteins (beans, lentils, tofu) and lean animal proteins (poultry, fish). Limit red and processed meats.
- **Using Herbs and Spices:** Turmeric, ginger, garlic, and cinnamon have anti-inflammatory properties and add flavor to meals without the need for excessive salt.
- **Staying Hydrated:** Drink plenty of water and incorporate herbal teas. Limit sugary drinks and alcohol.

STOCKING YOUR PANTRY AND KITCHEN ESSENTIALS

To set yourself up for success, stock your kitchen with these anti-inflammatory staples:

- **Fresh Produce:** Leafy greens (spinach, kale), berries (blueberries, strawberries), cruciferous vegetables (broccoli, cauliflower), and other colorful fruits and vegetables.
- **Whole Grains:** Quinoa, brown rice, oats, barley, and whole wheat products.
- **Healthy Fats:** Extra-virgin olive oil, avocado oil, coconut oil, nuts (almonds, walnuts), and seeds (chia, flax).
- **Proteins:** Legumes (lentils, chickpeas, black beans), nuts and seeds, tofu, tempeh, poultry, and fatty fish.
- **Herbs and Spices:** Fresh and dried herbs (parsley, cilantro, basil), spices (turmeric, ginger, cumin, cinnamon), garlic, and onions.
- **Beverages:** Herbal teas, green tea, coconut water, and plenty of filtered water.

KITCHEN TOOLS AND EQUIPMENT

Equipping your kitchen with the right tools makes preparing anti-inflammatory meals easier and more enjoyable:

- **Cutting Boards and Knives:** Invest in a good set of sharp knives and sturdy cutting boards.
- **Blender and Food Processor:** Essential for smoothies, soups, sauces, and dips.
- **Cookware:** Non-stick pans, a sturdy skillet, saucepans, and a stockpot.
- **Baking Sheets and Dishes:** For roasting vegetables and baking healthy treats.
- **Storage Containers:** Glass or BPA-free containers for meal prepping and storing leftovers.

TIPS FOR SUCCESS: MEAL PLANNING AND PREPARING

Planning your meals ahead of time helps ensure you stick to an anti-inflammatory diet and makes grocery shopping more efficient. Here are some strategies:

- **Weekly Meal Plans:** Spend some time each week planning your meals and snacks. Include a variety of foods to cover all essential nutrients.
- **Batch Cooking:** Prepare larger quantities of grains, legumes, and proteins that can be used in multiple meals throughout the week.
- **Utilize Leftovers:** Transform leftovers into new meals to save time and reduce waste. For example, roasted vegetables can be added to salads or grain bowls.

MEAL PREPPING TIPS

- Prep Ingredients in Advance: Wash and chop vegetables, cook grains, and prepare proteins in advance to streamline meal preparation during the week.
- Portion Control: Divide meals into individual portions to make it easier to grab and go.
- Storage: Use clear containers to easily see what's inside, and label them with the contents and date.

INCORPORATING ANTI-INFLAMMATORY FOODS INTO EVERYDAY MEALS

Here are some practical tips for incorporating anti-inflammatory foods into your daily diet:

- **Breakfast:** Start your day with a smoothie packed with berries, spinach, flaxseed, and almond milk. Alternatively, try overnight oats with chia seeds, nuts, and fresh fruit.
- **Lunch:** Opt for a large salad with a variety of colorful vegetables, lean protein (such as grilled chicken or chickpeas), and a drizzle of olive oil and lemon juice.
- **Dinner:** Focus on balanced meals that include a lean protein, a whole grain, and plenty of vegetables. For example, a quinoa bowl with roasted vegetables, grilled salmon, and a tahini dressing.
- Snacks: Keep healthy snacks on hand, such as a handful of nuts, sliced vegetables with hummus, or an apple with almond butter.

COOKING TECHNIQUES

Focus on cooking methods that preserve nutrients and reduce the formation of harmful substances:

- **Steaming and Grilling:** These methods help retain nutrients in vegetables and proteins.
- **Avoid Deep Frying:** Opt for baking, roasting, or air frying to minimize unhealthy fats.
- **Using Fresh Ingredients:** Whenever possible, use fresh, whole ingredients to maximize nutrient intake.

28-DAY MEAL PLAN

WEEK 1

	BREAKFAST	LUNCH	DINNER
DAY 1	Avocado and Smoked Salmon Toast	Chicken Caesar Salad	Chicken Alfredo with Zoodles
DAY 2	Greek Yogurt Parfait	Turkey Lettuce Wraps	Shrimp and Veggie Stir-Fry
DAY 3	Quinoa Breakfast Bowl	Tuna and White Bean Salad	Turkey and Quinoa Stuffed Peppers
DAY 4	Peanut Butter Banana Smoothie	Vegetable and Hummus Wrap	Baked Salmon with Quinoa and Asparagus
DAY 5	Oatmeal with Nuts and Berries	Chickpea and Avocado Sandwich	Beef and Broccoli
DAY 6	Egg and Veggie Scramble	Lentil and Vegetable Stew	Stuffed Bell Peppers
DAY 7	Sweet Potato Hash	Quinoa and Black Bean Salad	Chicken and Pesto Pasta

	BREAKFAST	LUNCH	DINNER
DAY 1	Green Smoothie	Zucchini Noodles with Pesto	Grilled Portobello Mushrooms
DAY 2	Chia Seed Pudding	Cabbage and Chicken Soup	Zoodle Pad Thai
DAY 3	Veggie Egg Muffins	Spinach and Feta Stuffed Mushrooms	Chicken Fajita Bowl
DAY 4	Protein-Packed Smoothie Bowl	Broccoli and Tofu Stir-Fry	Eggplant Parmesan
DAY 5	Cucumber and Tomato Salad	Cauliflower Fried Rice	Beef and Broccoli
DAY 6	Tofu Scramble	Greek Salad with Grilled Chicken	Salmon and Avocado Sushi Bowl
DAY 7	Sweet Potato Hash	Vegetable and Lentil Soup	Chicken and Veggie Kebabs

Repeat Week 1 and Week 2 to complete the 28-Day Meal Plan.
 Each week has a mix of lean proteins, complex carbohydrates, healthy fats, and fiber-rich foods to ensure optimal digestive health.

TURMERIC AND GINGER LATTE WITH ALMOND MILK

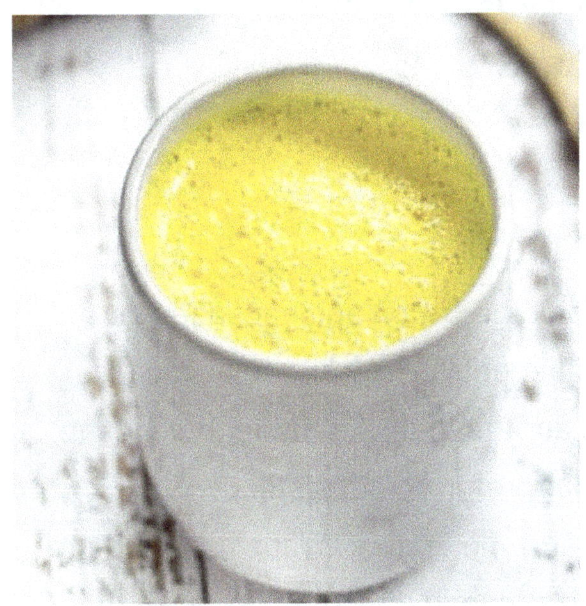

Cook Time: 5 Mins

Serving Size: 2

INGREDIENTS

- 2 cups unsweetened almond milk
- 1 teaspoon ground turmeric
- 1 teaspoon ground ginger
- 1/2 teaspoon ground cinnamon
- 1 tablespoon coconut oil (optional for creaminess)
- 1 tablespoon honey or maple syrup (adjust to taste)
- 1/2 teaspoon vanilla extract
- Pinch of black pepper (enhances turmeric absorption)
- A dash of nutmeg (optional, for extra flavor)

NUTRITIONAL FACTS

- Calories: 120kcal
- Carbohydrates: 10g | Protein: 1g
- Fat: 9g | Fiber: 2g | Sugar: 6g

INSTRUCTIONS

- In a small saucepan, heat the almond milk over medium heat until it starts to simmer. Do not let it boil.
- Reduce the heat to low and whisk in the turmeric, ginger, cinnamon, coconut oil, honey (or maple syrup), vanilla extract, and black pepper.
- Continue to whisk the mixture until all the ingredients are well combined and the milk is heated through (about 2-3 minutes).
- For a frothier latte, you can carefully transfer the mixture to a blender and blend for 30 seconds. Alternatively, use a handheld frother directly in the saucepan.
- Pour the latte into mugs. Sprinkle a dash of nutmeg on top if desired.
- Serve warm and enjoy the soothing, anti-inflammatory benefits of this golden latte.

KETO BREAKFAST BURRITO

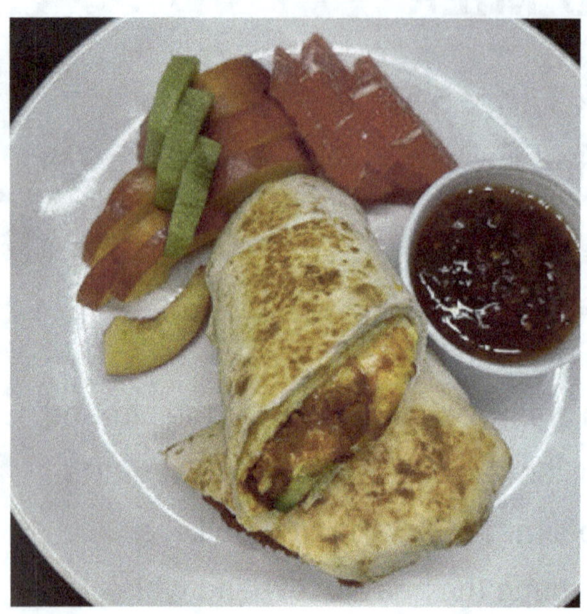

Cook Time: 20 Mins

Serving Size: 2

INSTRUCTIONS

- Cook the bacon and sausage in a skillet until crispy and fully cooked.
- In another pan, scramble the eggs to your preferred consistency.
- Warm the Egglife Wraps according to the package directions to make them flexible.
- Lay out the wraps and evenly distribute the scrambled eggs, bacon, and sausage onto each wrap.
- Add optional ingredients such as avocado or cheese if desired.
- Roll the wraps tightly, tucking in the ends as you roll.

INGREDIENTS

- 2 Original Egglife Wraps (Zero carbs)
- 2 Breakfast Chicken Sausage Links (Zero carbs)
- 2 strips of Thick Center-Cut Bacon
- 2 Large Eggs
- Optional toppings: Avocado, Cheese, Sour Cream, Sriracha, Zero Carb Cheese Sauce

NUTRITIONAL FACTS

- Calories: 300 kcal
- Carbohydrates: 0g net carbs
- Protein: High (exact amount depends on the type of sausage and bacon used)
- Fat: High

MISO SOUP WITH TOFU AND SEAWEED

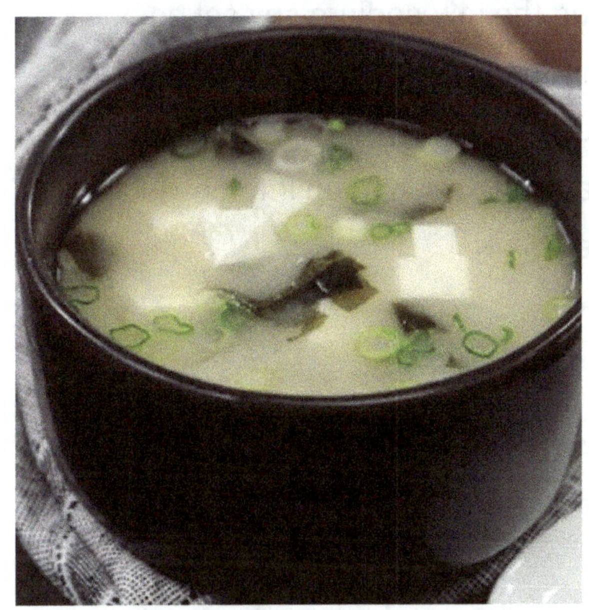

Cook Time: 15 Mins

Serving Size: 4

INGREDIENTS

- 4 cups water
- 1 cup dashi broth (use a kombu-based dashi for anti-inflammatory properties)
- 3 tablespoons miso paste (preferably white or yellow for a milder flavor)
- 1 cup firm tofu (cut into small cubes)
- 1/4 cup dried wakame seaweed (soaked in water for 10 minutes and drained)
- 1/4 cup green onions (thinly sliced)
- 1/2 cup mushrooms (shiitake or enoki, sliced)

INSTRUCTIONS

- If you're using dried kombu, soak a 4-inch piece in 4 cups of water for 30 minutes. Bring to a simmer over medium heat, then remove kombu before boiling.
- In a medium-sized pot, combine the water and dashi broth. Bring to a gentle simmer over medium heat.
- In a small bowl, mix the miso paste with a little hot water from the pot to dissolve it. Stir this mixture back into the pot. Ensure the heat is low to prevent boiling, as high heat can destroy the beneficial properties of miso.
- Gently add the cubed tofu and soaked, drained seaweed into the pot. Let it simmer for 2-3 minutes.
- Add the sliced mushrooms, green onions, and grated ginger (if using). Simmer for another 2-3 minutes until the mushrooms are tender.

INGREDIENTS

- 1 teaspoon grated ginger (optional, for added anti-inflammatory benefits)
- 1 tablespoon low-sodium soy sauce (or tamari for gluten-free option)

INGREDIENTS

- Calories: 80kcal
- Protein: 5g
- Carbohydrates: 7g
- Fat: 3g
- Fiber: 1g

INSTRUCTIONS

- Add the low-sodium soy sauce or tamari to taste. Adjust seasoning as needed.
- Ladle the miso soup into bowls and serve hot.

SARDINE AND AVOCADO TOAST

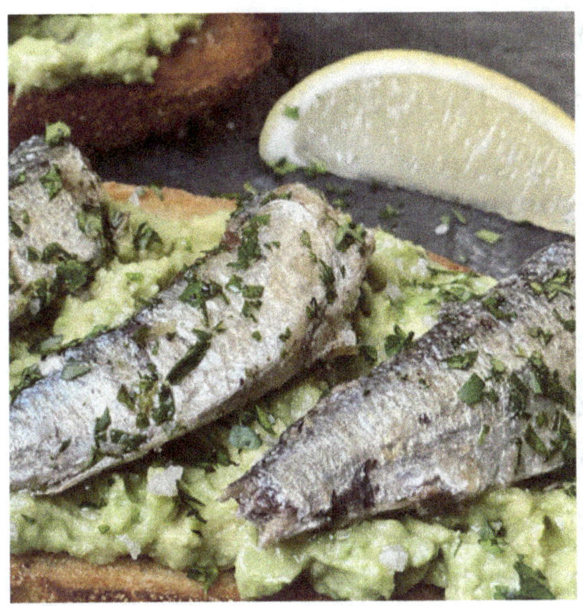

Cook Time: 5 Mins

Serving Size: 2

INGREDIENTS

- 2 slices of whole-grain or sourdough bread
- 1 ripe avocado
- 1 can (3.75 oz) of sardines in olive oil, drained
- 1 lemon
- 1 small clove of garlic, minced
- A handful of fresh cilantro or parsley, chopped
- 1 tablespoon of extra-virgin olive oil
- Sea salt, to taste
- Freshly ground black pepper, to taste
- A pinch of red pepper flakes (optional)
- Microgreens or arugula, for garnish (optional)

INSTRUCTIONS

- Toast Bread: Toast the bread until golden.
- Mash Avocado: Mash avocado with garlic, lemon juice, salt, and pepper.
- Spread: Spread mashed avocado on toasted bread.
- Top with Sardines: Place sardines on avocado spread.
- Garnish: Drizzle olive oil, sprinkle herbs, red pepper flakes, and microgreens.
- Serve: Enjoy immediately.

NUTRITIONAL FACTS

- Calories: 350
- Protein: 15g
- Carbs: 22g
- Fiber: 9g
- Sugars: 2g
- Fat: 24g

MATCHA GREEN TEA SMOOTHIE

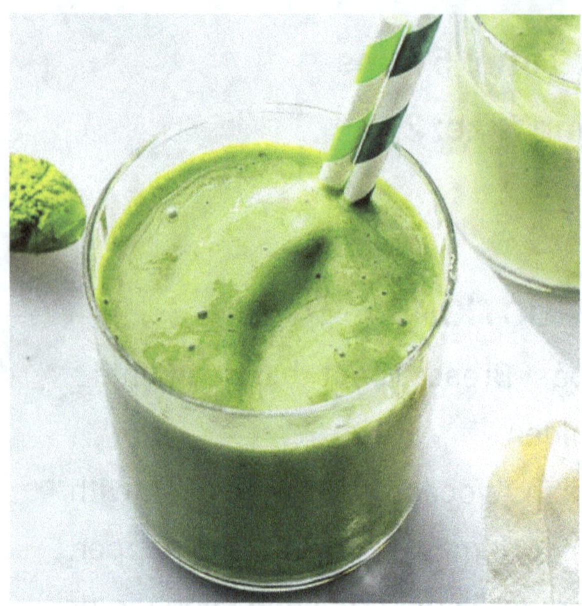

Prep Time: 5 Mins

Blending Time: 2 Mins

Serving Size: 1

INSTRUCTIONS

- Measure out all the ingredients. If you don't have frozen banana or pineapple chunks, you can use fresh ones but add more ice cubes to achieve the desired thickness.
- In a high-speed blender, combine the matcha green tea powder, almond milk, frozen banana, frozen pineapple chunks, baby spinach, chia seeds, ground turmeric, ground ginger, and honey or maple syrup if using.
- If you prefer a thicker, colder smoothie, add the ice cubes.
- Blend all the ingredients on high speed until smooth and creamy. This should take about 1-2 minutes.
- Pour the smoothie into a glass and enjoy immediately.

INGREDIENTS

- 1 teaspoon matcha green tea powder
- 1 cup unsweetened almond milk (or any plant-based milk)
- 1 frozen banana
- 1/2 cup frozen pineapple chunks
- 1/2 cup baby spinach
- 1 tablespoon chia seeds
- 1/2 teaspoon ground turmeric
- 1/2 teaspoon ground ginger
- 1 teaspoon honey or maple syrup (optional, for sweetness)
- 1/2 cup ice cubes (optional, for a thicker smoothie)

NUTRITIONAL FACTS

- Calories: 280kcal | Fat: 10g
- Carbohydrates: 43g | Fiber: 6g
- Sugars: 10g
- Protein: 7g

TOFU SCRAMBLE

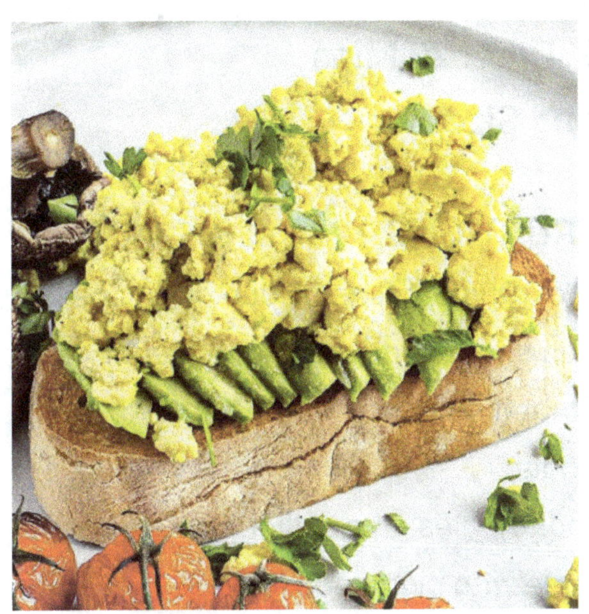

Cook Time: 15

Serving Size: 2

INGREDIENTS

- 1 block of firm tofu, drained and crumbled
- 1 tablespoon olive oil
- 1 small onion, diced
- 1 bell pepper, diced
- 2 cloves garlic, minced
- 1 teaspoon turmeric
- 1/2 teaspoon cumin
- Salt and pepper to taste
- Optional toppings: diced tomatoes, avocado slices, chopped cilantro

INSTRUCTIONS

- Heat olive oil in a large skillet over medium heat.
- Add diced onion and bell pepper to the skillet and sauté until softened, about 5 minutes.
- Add minced garlic to the skillet and cook for an additional minute.
- Add crumbled tofu to the skillet, along with turmeric, cumin, salt, and pepper. Stir well to combine.
- Cook the tofu mixture for about 5-7 minutes, stirring occasionally, until heated through and slightly browned.
- Taste and adjust seasoning if necessary.
- Serve hot with optional toppings if desired.

NUTRITIONAL FACTS

- Calories: 210kcal | Fat: 14g
- Total Carbohydrates: 10g
- Fiber: 3g | Sugars: 4g
- Protein: 16g

CINNAMON AND APPLE QUINOA

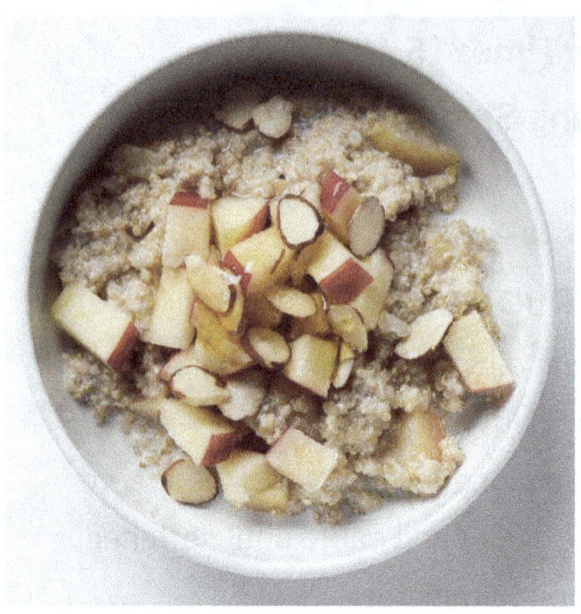

Cook Time: 20 Mins

Serving Size: 4

INSTRUCTIONS

- Cook Quinoa: Rinse 1 cup of quinoa, then simmer in 2 cups of water or almond milk for 15 minutes until tender.
- Cook Apples: In a skillet, sauté diced apple with cinnamon, ginger, turmeric, and nutmeg until tender (5-7 mins).
- Combine: Mix cooked apples with cooked quinoa. Add maple syrup or honey (optional), nuts, raisins, vanilla, and a pinch of salt.
- Serve: Divide into bowls and garnish with mint leaves if desired.

INGREDIENTS

- 1 cup quinoa, rinsed
- 2 cups water or unsweetened almond milk
- 1 large apple, peeled, cored, and diced
- 1 teaspoon ground cinnamon
- 1/2 teaspoon ground ginger
- 1/4 teaspoon ground turmeric
- 1/4 teaspoon ground nutmeg
- 1 tablespoon pure maple syrup or honey (optional)
- 1/4 cup chopped walnuts or pecans
- 1/4 cup raisins or dried cranberries (unsweetened)
- 1 teaspoon vanilla extract
- Pinch of sea salt
- Fresh mint leaves for garnish (optional)

NUTRITIONAL FACTS

- Calories: 250
- Protein: 6g
- Fat: 8g
- Carbohydrates: 40g
- Fiber: 6g
- Sugars: 12g

BERRY AND FLAXSEED MUFFINS

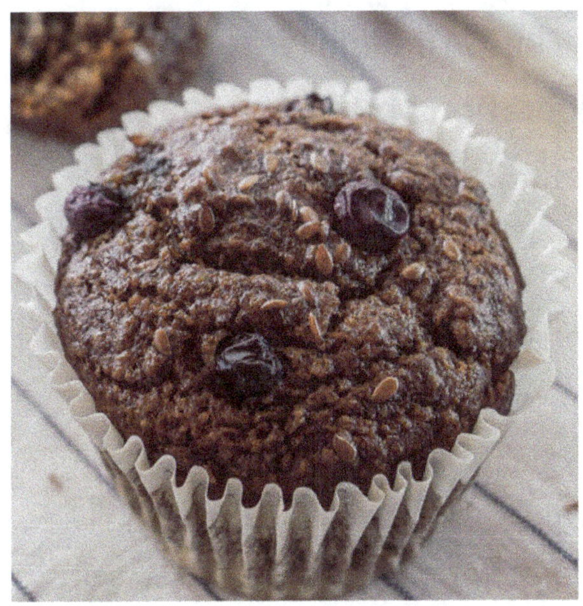

Cook Time: 22 Mins

Serving Size: 12

INGREDIENTS

- 1 cup whole wheat flour
- 1 cup almond flour
- 1/2 cup ground flaxseed
- 1 teaspoon baking powder
- 1/2 teaspoon baking soda
- 1/4 teaspoon salt
- 2 large eggs
- 1/2 cup unsweetened applesauce
- 1/4 cup honey or maple syrup
- 1/4 cup olive oil or melted coconut oil
- 1 teaspoon vanilla extract
- 1 cup mixed berries (such as blueberries, raspberries, and strawberries), fresh or frozen

INSTRUCTIONS

- Preheat oven to 350°F (175°C). Prepare a muffin tin with liners or grease.
- In a large bowl, mix whole wheat flour, almond flour, flaxseed, baking powder, baking soda, and salt.
- In another bowl, beat eggs and combine with applesauce, honey, oil, and vanilla.
- Add wet ingredients to dry ingredients and stir until just combined.
- Fold in berries.
- Fill muffin cups 3/4 full and bake for 18-22 minutes.
- Cool in tin for 5 minutes, then transfer to a wire rack.

NUTRITIONAL FACTS

- Calories: 180kcal | Total Fat: 10g
- Carbohydrates: 19g | Fiber: 4g
- Sugars: 8g | Protein: 5g

PUMPKIN SPICE CHIA PUDDING

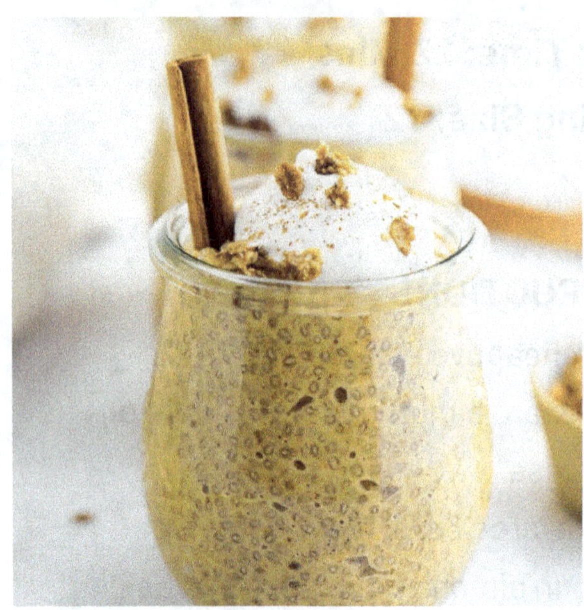

INGREDIENTS

- 1 cup unsweetened almond milk (or any other plant-based milk)
- 1/2 cup pumpkin puree
- 1/4 cup chia seeds
- 1-2 tablespoons maple syrup (adjust to taste)
- 1 teaspoon vanilla extract
- 1 teaspoon ground cinnamon
- 1/2 teaspoon ground ginger
- 1/4 teaspoon ground nutmeg
- 1/4 teaspoon ground cloves
- A pinch of sea salt
- Optional toppings: chopped nuts, shredded coconut, fresh berries

NUTRITIONAL FACTS

- Calories: 140 kcal | Protein: 4g
- Carbohydrates: 18 g | Fiber: 8 g
- Sugars: 6g | Fat: 7g

Prep Time: 10 Mins

Refrigeration: 4 Hours

Serving Size: 4

INSTRUCTIONS

- In a medium bowl, combine the almond milk, pumpkin puree, maple syrup, vanilla extract, cinnamon, ginger, nutmeg, cloves, and sea salt. Whisk until smooth and well combined.
- Add the chia seeds to the mixture and stir well to ensure the seeds are evenly distributed. Let the mixture sit for about 10 minutes, then stir again to prevent the seeds from clumping together.
- Cover the bowl and refrigerate for at least 4 hours, or overnight, until the chia seeds have absorbed the liquid and the mixture has thickened to a pudding-like consistency.
- Stir the pudding well before serving. Divide into individual serving bowls or jars. Add your favorite toppings, such as chopped nuts, shredded coconut, or fresh berries.

BANANA AND WALNUT SMOOTHIE

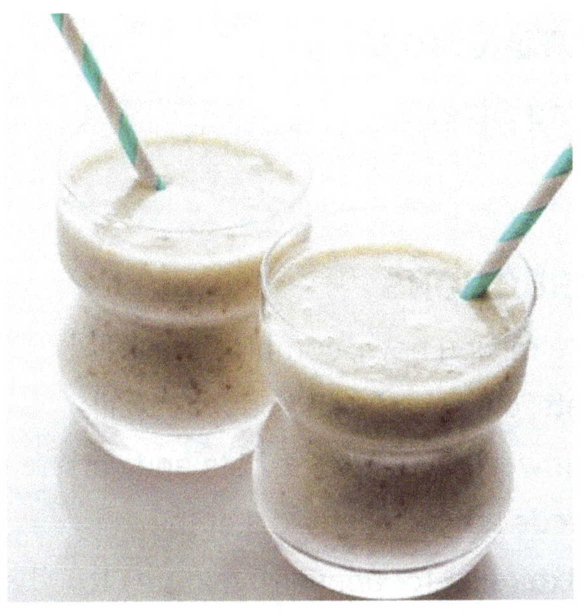

Prep Time: 5 Mins

Blend Time: 2 Mins

Serving Size: 2

INSTRUCTIONS

- **Prepare Ingredients:** Peel and slice the banana. Measure out the walnuts, almond milk, Greek yogurt, ground flaxseeds, turmeric powder, cinnamon, and honey or maple syrup if using.
- **Blend Smoothie:** Place all ingredients, including the ice cubes, into a high-speed blender.
- **Blend:** Blend on high speed until smooth and creamy. This should take about 1-2 minutes, depending on the strength of your blender.
- **Serve:** Pour the smoothie into a glass. Enjoy immediately.

INGREDIENTS

- 1 large banana, peeled and sliced
- 1/2 cup raw walnuts
- 1 cup unsweetened almond milk (or any plant-based milk)
- 1/2 cup plain Greek yogurt (or a dairy-free yogurt alternative)
- 1 tablespoon ground flaxseeds
- 1 teaspoon turmeric powder
- 1/2 teaspoon cinnamon
- 1 teaspoon honey or maple syrup (optional, for added sweetness)
- 1/2 cup ice cubes

NUTRITIONAL FACTS

- Calories: 285 kcal
- Protein: 8g | Fat: 19g
- Saturated Fat: 1.5g
- Carbohydrates: 23g
- Fiber: 5g
- Sugars: 12g

TROPICAL CHIA-OAT CEREAL BOWL

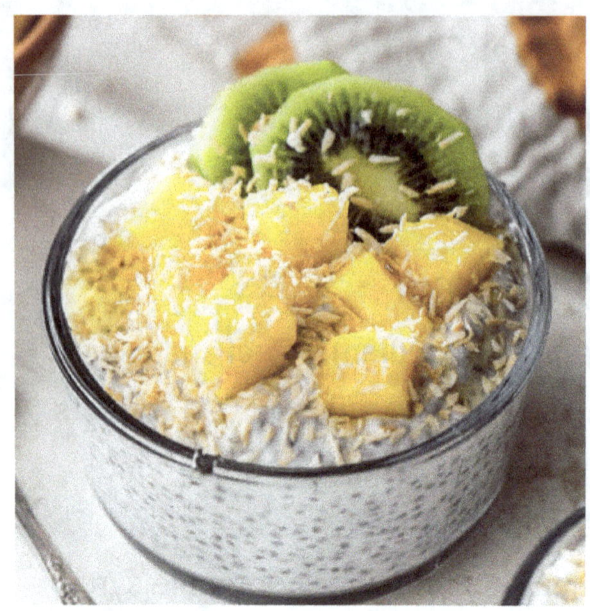

Cook Time: 10 Mins

Serving Size: 2

INGREDIENTS

- 1/4 cup rolled oats
- 2 tablespoons chia seeds
- 1/2 cup coconut milk (unsweetened)
- 1/2 cup diced pineapple
- 1/2 cup diced mango
- 1 tablespoon shredded coconut (unsweetened)
- 1 tablespoon honey or maple syrup (optional, for sweetness)
- A handful of mixed berries (optional, for garnish)
- A sprinkle of ground turmeric (optional, for anti-inflammatory benefits)
- A sprinkle of ground cinnamon (optional, for flavor)

INSTRUCTIONS

- In a mixing bowl, combine the rolled oats, chia seeds, and coconut milk.
- Stir well to ensure the oats and chia seeds are fully coated. Let the mixture sit for about 10 minutes to allow the chia seeds to gel and the oats to soften.
- After 10 minutes, stir in the diced pineapple, diced mango, and shredded coconut. If desired, add honey or maple syrup for sweetness, and sprinkle with ground turmeric and cinnamon for flavor and anti-inflammatory benefits.
- Transfer the mixture into serving bowls.
- Top each bowl with a handful of mixed berries for extra flavor and nutrition.
- Serve immediately and enjoy!

ROASTED VEGETABLE SALAD WITH QUINOA

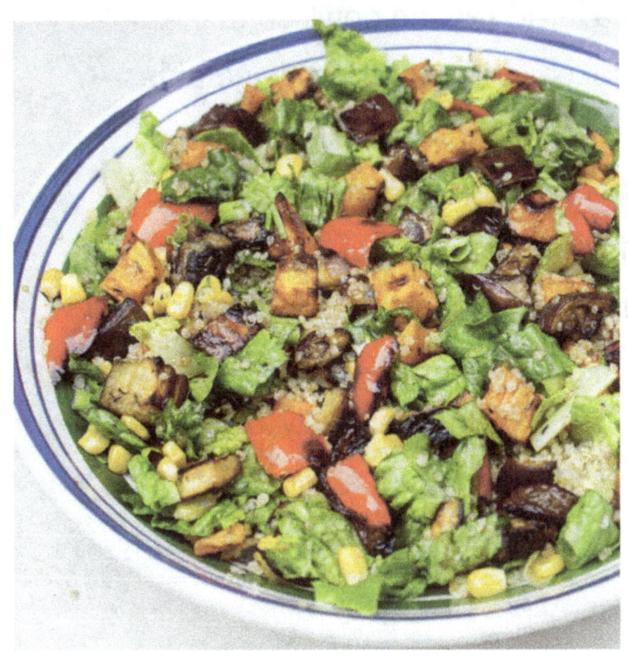

Cook Time: 20 Mins

Serving Size: 4

INGREDIENTS

- 1 cup quinoa, rinsed
- 2 cups water
- 2 cups mixed vegetables (such as bell peppers, zucchini, cherry tomatoes, red onion, carrots), chopped
- 2 tablespoons olive oil
- 1 teaspoon dried herbs (such as thyme, rosemary, oregano)
- Salt and pepper to taste
- 2 cups baby spinach or mixed greens
- 1/4 cup chopped fresh parsley
- 1/4 cup chopped walnuts or almonds (optional)

INSTRUCTIONS

- Preheat the oven to 400°F (200°C).
- In a saucepan, combine quinoa and water. Bring to a boil, then reduce heat to low, cover, and simmer for 15-20 minutes, or until quinoa is cooked and water is absorbed. Remove from heat and let it sit, covered, for 5 minutes. Fluff with a fork and set aside.
- In a large bowl, toss mixed vegetables with olive oil, dried herbs, salt, and pepper until evenly coated. Spread the vegetables in a single layer on a baking sheet.
- Roast the vegetables in the preheated oven for 20-25 minutes, or until they are tender and slightly caramelized, stirring halfway through cooking.
- In a small bowl, whisk together the ingredients for the dressing: olive oil, balsamic vinegar, minced garlic, Dijon mustard, salt, and pepper.

INGREDIENTS

For the dressing:

- 3 tablespoons extra virgin olive oil
- 2 tablespoons balsamic vinegar
- 1 clove garlic, minced
- 1 teaspoon Dijon mustard
- Salt and pepper to taste

NUTRITIONAL FACTS

- Calories: 320
- Total Fat: 18g
- Total Carbohydrates: 35g
- Dietary Fiber: 7g
- Sugars: 4g
- Protein: 8g

INSTRUCTIONS

- In a large serving bowl, combine cooked quinoa, roasted vegetables, baby spinach or mixed greens, chopped parsley, and chopped nuts (if using). Drizzle with the prepared dressing and toss gently to combine.
- Serve the roasted vegetable salad with quinoa immediately, or chill in the refrigerator for a couple of hours before serving for enhanced flavors.

GRILLED ASPARAGUS

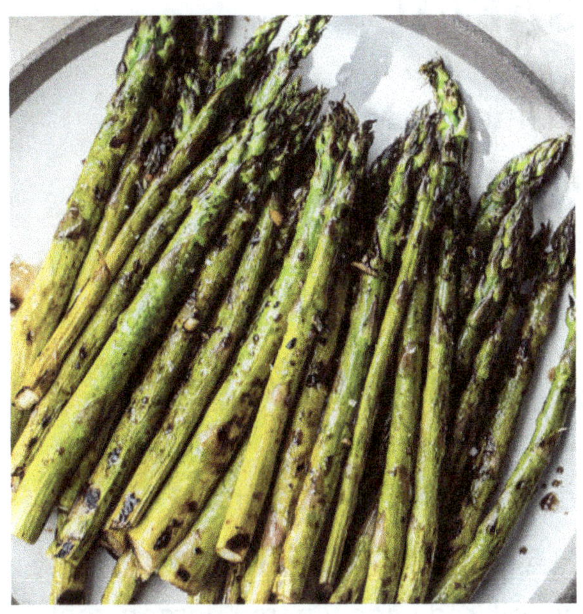

INSTRUCTIONS

- Preheat Grill: Preheat your grill to medium-high heat (about 400°F or 200°C).
- Prepare Asparagus: Wash the asparagus and trim the tough ends off the bottom of the spears.
- Season Asparagus: In a large bowl, toss the asparagus with the olive oil, lemon zest, lemon juice, minced garlic, sea salt, and black pepper until evenly coated.
- Grill Asparagus: Place the asparagus spears directly on the grill grates, perpendicular to the grates to prevent them from falling through. Grill for 5-7 minutes, turning occasionally, until tender and lightly charred.
- Serve: Remove the asparagus from the grill and transfer to a serving plate. Sprinkle with chopped fresh parsley if desired. Serve immediately.

INGREDIENTS

- 1 pound fresh asparagus spears, trimmed
- 2 tablespoons extra virgin olive oil
- 1 teaspoon lemon zest
- 1 tablespoon fresh lemon juice
- 1 clove garlic, minced
- 1/2 teaspoon sea salt
- 1/4 teaspoon black pepper
- 1 tablespoon fresh parsley, chopped (optional)

NUTRITIONAL FACTS

- Calories: 60kcal | Fat: 5g
- Carbohydrates: 5g
- Fiber: 2.5g
- Sugars: 2g
- Protein: 2.5g

MEDITERRANEAN TUNA AND WHITE BEAN SALAD

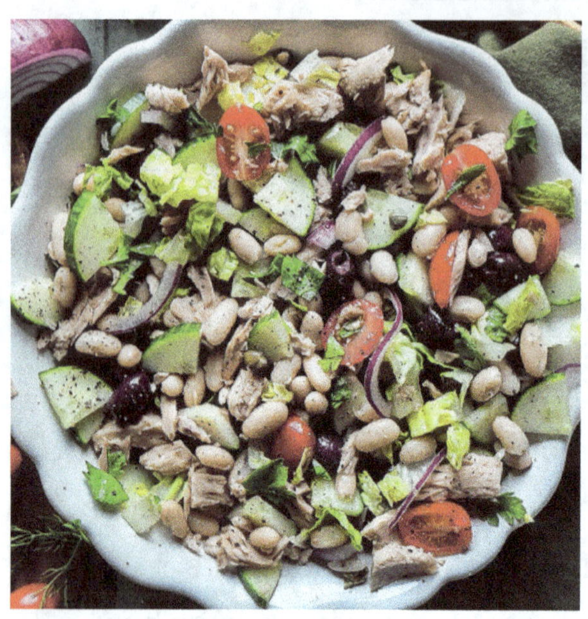

Cook Time: 15 Mins

Serving Size: 2

INSTRUCTIONS

- In a large bowl, combine the drained tuna, white beans, cherry tomatoes, red onion, olives, and parsley.
- In a small bowl, whisk together the olive oil, red wine vinegar, lemon zest, salt, and pepper.
- Pour the dressing over the salad and toss gently to combine.
- Serve the salad over a bed of mixed greens.

INGREDIENTS

- 1 can (5 oz) tuna packed in water, drained
- 1 can (15 oz) white beans (cannellini or navy beans), drained and rinsed
- 1 cup cherry tomatoes, halved
- 1/2 cup red onion, finely chopped
- 1/4 cup kalamata olives, pitted and sliced
- 1/4 cup fresh parsley, chopped
- 2 cups mixed greens (arugula, spinach, or your choice)
- 2 tbsp extra virgin olive oil
- 1 tbsp red wine vinegar
- 1 tsp lemon zest
- Salt and pepper to taste

NUTRITIONAL FACTS

- Calories: 350kcal
- Protein: 25g
- Carbohydrates: 30g
- Fat: 15g
- Fiber: 8g

MASON JAR POWER SALAD WITH CHICKPEAS & TUNA

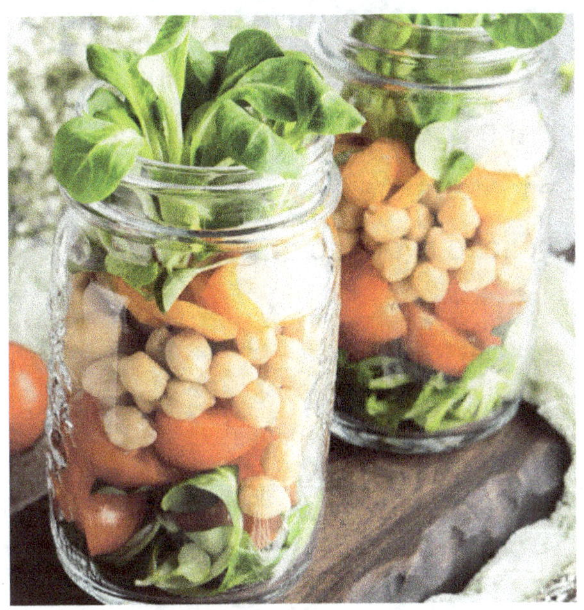

Prep Time: 20 Mins

Serving Size: 4

INSTRUCTIONS

Prepare the Dressing:

- In a small bowl or jar, whisk together the olive oil, lemon juice, minced garlic, Dijon mustard, honey (or maple syrup), salt, and pepper until well combined.

Assemble the Salad in Mason Jars:

- Divide the dressing evenly among 4 large mason jars, pouring it into the bottom of each jar.

Layer the salad ingredients in the following order:

- Chickpeas
- Tuna
- Cherry tomatoes
- Cucumber
- Red onion
- Kalamata olives
- Feta cheese
- Mixed greens
- Seal the jars with lids and refrigerate until ready to serve.

INGREDIENTS

For the Salad:

- 1 cup canned chickpeas, drained and rinsed
- 1 can (5 oz) tuna packed in water, drained
- 1 cup cherry tomatoes, halved
- 1 cup cucumber, diced
- 1/4 cup red onion, finely chopped
- 1/4 cup Kalamata olives, pitted and halved
- 1/2 cup feta cheese, crumbled
- 2 cups mixed greens (spinach, arugula, kale)
- 1 avocado, sliced (add just before serving to prevent browning)

INGREDIENTS

For the Dressing:

- 1/4 cup extra-virgin olive oil
- 2 tablespoons lemon juice (freshly squeezed)
- 1 clove garlic, minced
- 1 teaspoon Dijon mustard
- 1 teaspoon honey or maple syrup
- Salt and pepper to taste

NUTRITIONAL FACTS

- Calories: 400 kcal
- Total Fat: 24g
- Carbohydrates: 24g
- Dietary Fiber: 7g
- Sugars: 6g
- Protein: 22g

INSTRUCTIONS

Serve the Salad:

- When ready to eat, give the jar a good shake to distribute the dressing, or pour the contents into a bowl and toss to combine.
- Add sliced avocado on top before serving.

CHICKPEA SALAD SANDWICH

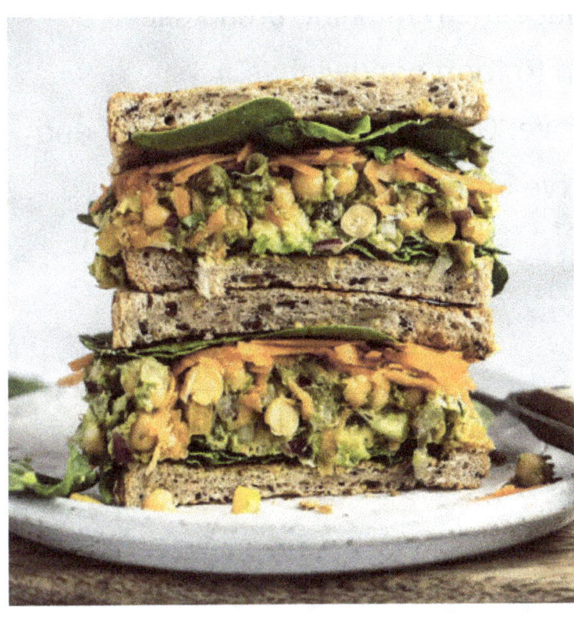

Prep Time: 15 Mins

Serving Size: 4

INSTRUCTIONS

- **Mash the Chickpeas:** In a medium bowl, use a fork or potato masher to mash the chickpeas. Leave some chunks for texture.
- **Prepare the Dressing:** In a small bowl, whisk together the Greek yogurt, olive oil, lemon juice, Dijon mustard, turmeric powder, ground cumin, black pepper, and salt (if using).
- **Combine Ingredients:** Add the chopped celery, grated carrot, red onion, and parsley to the mashed chickpeas. Pour the dressing over the mixture and stir until well combined.
- **Assemble the Sandwiches:** Toast the bread slices if desired. Spread a generous amount of the chickpea salad on four slices of bread. Top with avocado slices and optional leafy greens or tomato slices.

INGREDIENTS

- 1 can (15 oz) chickpeas, drained and rinsed
- 1/4 cup plain Greek yogurt (non-fat or low-fat)
- 1 tbsp extra virgin olive oil
- 1 tbsp lemon juice
- 1 tsp Dijon mustard
- 1/2 tsp turmeric powder
- 1/2 tsp ground cumin
- 1/4 tsp black pepper
- 1/4 tsp salt (optional)
- 1 small celery stalk, finely chopped
- 1 small carrot, grated
- 2 tbsp red onion, finely chopped
- 2 tbsp fresh parsley, chopped

INGREDIENTS

- 1 small avocado, sliced
- 8 slices of whole grain or gluten-free bread
- Optional: leafy greens (such as spinach or arugula), tomato slices

NUTRITIONAL FACTS

- Calories: 350 kcal
- Protein: 12g
- Carbohydrates: 50g
- Dietary Fiber: 10g
- Total Fat: 12g
- Saturated Fat: 2g
- Cholesterol: 5mg
- Sodium: 400mg (can vary based on added salt and bread type)
- Sugars: 5g

INSTRUCTIONS

- Place the remaining bread slices on top to form sandwiches.
- **Serve:** Cut the sandwiches in half and serve immediately.

FISH EN PAPILLOTE

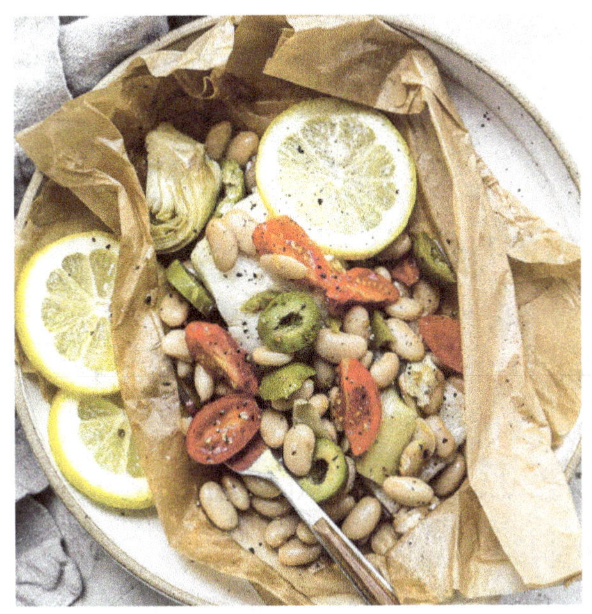

INGREDIENTS

- 4 fillets of white fish (such as cod, halibut, or tilapia), about 6 oz each
- 1 small zucchini, thinly sliced
- 1 small yellow squash, thinly sliced
- 1 red bell pepper, thinly sliced
- 1 carrot, julienned
- 1 lemon, thinly sliced
- 4 sprigs of fresh thyme
- 2 tablespoons extra-virgin olive oil
- 4 cloves garlic, minced
- 1 teaspoon fresh ginger, minced
- 1 teaspoon turmeric powder
- Salt and pepper to taste
- 4 sheets of parchment paper (about 15 inches square)

Cook Time: 20 Mins

Serving Size: 4

INSTRUCTIONS

- Preheat oven to 400°F (200°C).
- Prepare parchment paper by folding each sheet in half.
- Assemble packets: Place a fish fillet on one half of each sheet, surround with vegetables, and top with garlic, ginger, turmeric, thyme, lemon, olive oil, salt, and pepper.
- Seal packets by folding and crimping edges tightly.
- Bake on a baking sheet for 20 minutes.
- Serve by transferring packets to plates and carefully opening.

NUTRITIONAL FACTS

- Calories: 250kcal
- Protein: 28g
- Carbohydrates: 10g
- Fat: 12g
- Fiber: 3g
- Sugar: 5g

BAKED STEELHEAD TROUT

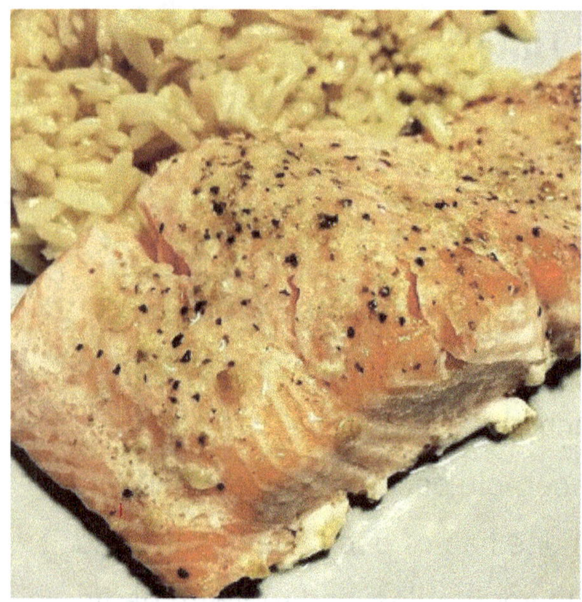

INGREDIENTS

- 1 lb steelhead trout fillet
- 2 tablespoons extra virgin olive oil
- 2 cloves garlic, minced
- 1 tablespoon fresh lemon juice
- 1 teaspoon lemon zest
- 1 tablespoon fresh dill, chopped
- 1 tablespoon fresh parsley, chopped
- 1 teaspoon ground turmeric
- 1/2 teaspoon ground black pepper
- 1/2 teaspoon sea salt
- 1 cup cherry tomatoes, halved
- 1 small red onion, thinly sliced

NUTRITIONAL FACTS

- Calories: 350 kcal | Protein: 35g
- Fat: 20g | Carbohydrates: 8g
- Fiber: 2g | Sugar: 4g

Cook Time: 25 Mins

Serving Size: 2

INSTRUCTIONS

- Preheat your oven to 375°F (190°C).
- Lightly grease a baking dish with a small amount of olive oil.
- Place the steelhead trout fillet in the baking dish.
- In a small bowl, mix together the olive oil, minced garlic, lemon juice, lemon zest, dill, parsley, turmeric, black pepper, and sea salt.
- Brush the mixture evenly over the trout fillet.
- Scatter the halved cherry tomatoes and sliced red onion around the trout in the baking dish.
- Place the baking dish in the preheated oven.
- Bake for about 20-25 minutes, or until the trout flakes easily with a fork and is opaque in the center.
- Remove from the oven and let it rest for a few minutes.
- Serve the baked steelhead trout with the roasted cherry tomatoes and red onions on the side.

ITALIAN SHRIMP SALAD

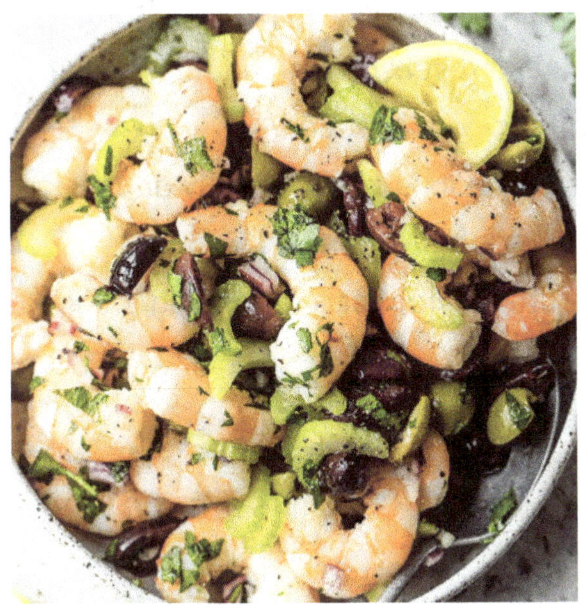

Cook Time: 8 Mins

Serving Size: 4

INSTRUCTIONS

- Heat 1 tablespoon of olive oil in a large skillet over medium heat.
- Add the minced garlic and red pepper flakes (if using) and sauté for about 1 minute until fragrant.
- Add the shrimp to the skillet and cook for 2-3 minutes on each side until they turn pink and opaque.
- Remove the shrimp from the skillet and let them cool slightly.
- In a large salad bowl, combine the cherry tomatoes, cucumber, red onion, kalamata olives, basil leaves, parsley, and mixed greens.
- In a small bowl, whisk together the 3 tablespoons of olive oil, apple cider vinegar, Dijon mustard, minced garlic, dried oregano, salt, and pepper.
- Add the cooked shrimp to the salad bowl.
- Drizzle the dressing over the salad and toss gently to combine.

INGREDIENTS

- 1 lb large shrimp, peeled and deveined
- 1 tbsp extra virgin olive oil
- 2 cloves garlic, minced
- 1/2 tsp red pepper flakes (optional for heat)
- 1/2 cup cherry tomatoes, halved
- 1 small cucumber, diced
- 1/4 red onion, thinly sliced
- 1/4 cup kalamata olives, pitted and sliced
- 1/4 cup fresh basil leaves, torn
- 1/4 cup fresh parsley, chopped
- 2 cups mixed greens (e.g., arugula, spinach, or a mix)
- 1 lemon, juiced
- Salt and freshly ground black pepper, to taste

INGREDIENTS

Dressing:

- 3 tbsp extra virgin olive oil
- 1 tbsp apple cider vinegar
- 1 tsp Dijon mustard
- 1 clove garlic, minced
- 1/2 tsp dried oregano
- Salt and freshly ground black pepper, to taste

NUTRITIONAL FACTS

- Calories: 240kcal
- Protein: 20g
- Carbohydrates: 8g
- Dietary Fiber: 3g
- Sugars: 3g
- Fat: 15g

INSTRUCTIONS

- Squeeze fresh lemon juice over the salad and season with additional salt and pepper, if needed.
- Serve the salad immediately or chill in the refrigerator for 10-15 minutes before serving for a refreshing touch.

THAI RED VEGETABLE CURRY

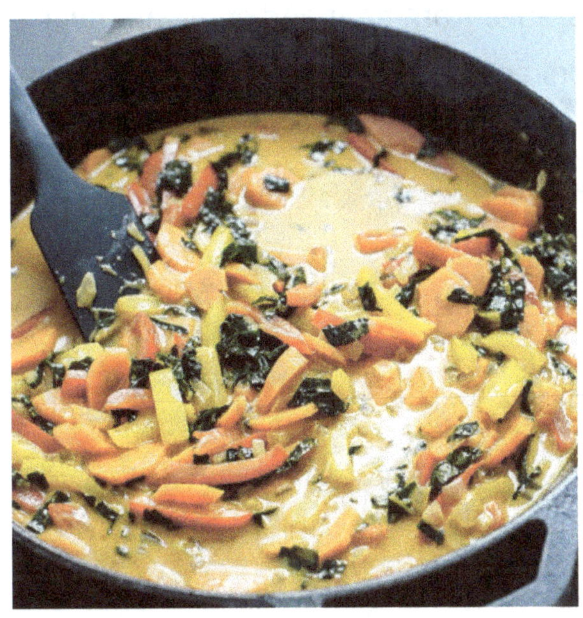

Cook Time: 20 Mins

Serving Size: 4

INGREDIENTS

- 2 tablespoons red curry paste (check for one without added sugar)
- 1 can (14 ounces) coconut milk (full-fat for creaminess)
- 1 cup vegetable broth
- 2 tablespoons coconut oil
- 2 cups mixed vegetables (such as bell peppers, broccoli, carrots, and snap peas)
- 1 small onion, sliced
- 3 cloves garlic, minced
- 1 tablespoon fresh ginger, grated
- 1 tablespoon tamari or soy sauce (low-sodium)
- 1 tablespoon maple syrup or honey (optional, adjust to taste)

INSTRUCTIONS

- Heat coconut oil in a large skillet or pot over medium heat. Add sliced onion and cook until softened, about 3-4 minutes.
- Stir in minced garlic and grated ginger, and cook for another 1-2 minutes until fragrant.
- Add the red curry paste to the skillet and cook for 1 minute, stirring constantly.
- Pour in the coconut milk and vegetable broth, stirring to combine. Bring the mixture to a simmer.
- Add mixed vegetables to the skillet and cook until they are tender but still crisp, about 5-7 minutes.
- Stir in tamari or soy sauce, and maple syrup or honey if using. Season with salt and pepper to taste.
- Let the curry simmer for another 2-3 minutes to allow the flavors to meld together.

INGREDIENTS

- Salt and pepper to taste
- Fresh cilantro leaves, for garnish
- Cooked rice or quinoa, for serving.

NUTRITIONAL FACTS

- Calories: 250
- Total Fat: 20g
- Total Carbohydrates: 18g
- Dietary Fiber: 4g
- Sugars: 6g
- Protein: 3g

INSTRUCTIONS

- Remove from heat and serve hot over cooked rice or quinoa.
- Garnish with fresh cilantro leaves before serving

MEDITERRANEAN SHEET PAN SALMON

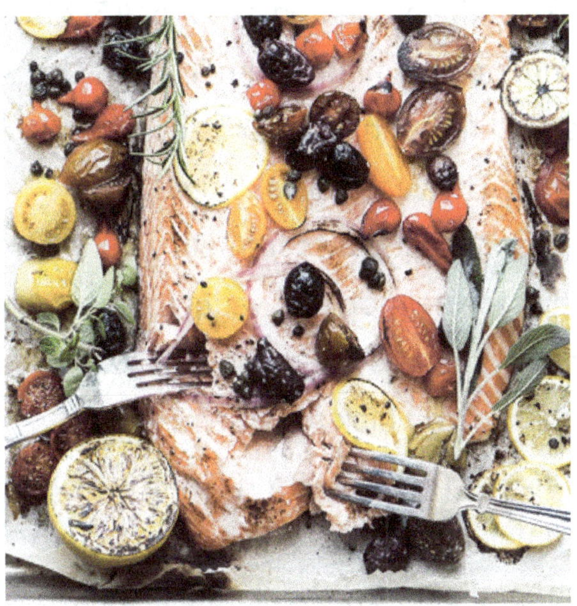

Cook Time: 20 Mins

Serving Size: 4

INSTRUCTIONS

- Preheat your oven to 400°F (200°C). Line a large baking sheet with parchment paper for easy cleanup.
- On the prepared baking sheet, arrange the red bell pepper, yellow bell pepper, red onion, zucchini, cherry tomatoes, and Kalamata olives.
- Drizzle the vegetables with 2 tablespoons of extra virgin olive oil and season with dried oregano, dried thyme, garlic powder, salt, and black pepper. Toss to coat the vegetables evenly.
- Move the vegetables to the sides of the baking sheet to make space in the center for the salmon fillets.
- Place the salmon fillets skin-side down on the baking sheet. Season the salmon with a pinch of salt and black pepper.

INGREDIENTS

For the Salmon and Vegetables:

- 4 salmon fillets (about 6 ounces each)
- 1 large red bell pepper, sliced into strips
- 1 large yellow bell pepper, sliced into strips
- 1 red onion, cut into wedges
- 1 zucchini, sliced into rounds
- 1 cup cherry tomatoes, halved
- 1/4 cup Kalamata olives, pitted and halved
- 2 tablespoons extra virgin olive oil
- 1 teaspoon dried oregano
- 1 teaspoon dried thyme
- 1 teaspoon garlic powder
- Salt and black pepper to taste

INGREDIENTS

- 8 oz whole wheat pasta
- 2 boneless, skinless chicken breasts, thinly sliced
- 2 tablespoons olive oil
- 2 cloves garlic, minced
- 1 cup cherry tomatoes, halved
- 2 cups spinach leaves
- ¼ cup basil pesto
- Salt and pepper to taste
- Grated Parmesan cheese for garnish (optional)

NUTRITIONAL FACTS

- Calories: 380
- Protein: 34g
- Total Fat: 22g
- Carbohydrates: 12g
- Dietary Fiber: 4g
- Sugars: 6g

INSTRUCTIONS

- Bake in the preheated oven for 15-20 minutes, or until the salmon is cooked through and flakes easily with a fork. The vegetables should be tender and slightly caramelized.
- While the salmon and vegetables are baking, prepare the dressing. In a small bowl, whisk together 2 tablespoons of extra virgin olive oil, lemon juice and zest, minced garlic, chopped parsley, chopped dill, Dijon mustard, salt, and black pepper.
- Once the salmon and vegetables are done, remove the baking sheet from the oven. Drizzle the lemon herb dressing over the salmon and vegetables.
- Serve immediately, garnished with additional fresh herbs if desired.

SOY GINGER SALMON

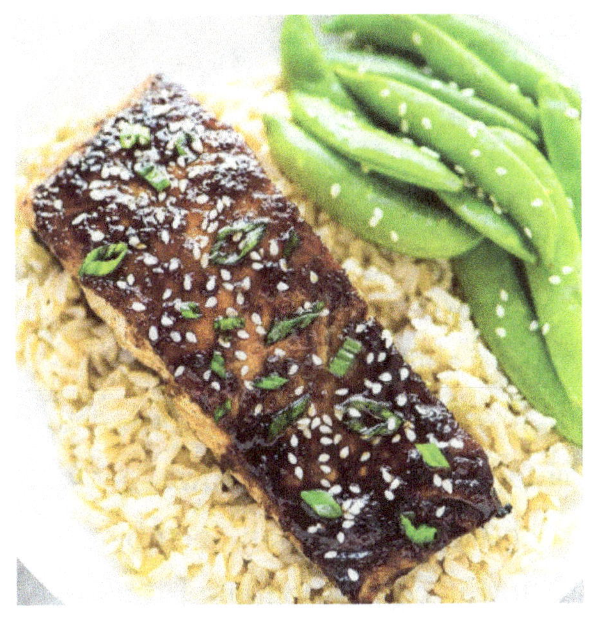

Cook Time: 15 Mins

Serving Size: 4

INGREDIENTS

For the Marinade:

- 1/4 cup low-sodium soy sauce or tamari (gluten-free)
- 2 tablespoons fresh ginger, grated
- 2 tablespoons honey or maple syrup
- 2 tablespoons fresh lime juice
- 2 cloves garlic, minced
- 1 tablespoon sesame oil
- 1 tablespoon rice vinegar

For the Salmon:

- 4 (6-ounce) wild-caught salmon fillets
- 2 tablespoons olive oil or avocado oil
- 1 tablespoon sesame seeds
- 2 green onions, thinly sliced

INSTRUCTIONS

- Whisk together marinade ingredients. Pour over salmon fillets in a dish or bag. Marinate in the fridge for 30 minutes to 2 hours.
- Preheat oven to 400°F (200°C).
- Place salmon on a greased or parchment-lined baking sheet.
- Drizzle with olive oil. Bake for 12-15 minutes until cooked through.
- Garnish with sesame seeds and green onions.
- Serve with steamed vegetables or a salad.

NUTRITIONAL FACTS

- Calories: 350kcal
- Protein: 30g
- Carbs: 12g (8g sugars)
- Fat: 20g (3g saturated, high in omega-3)
- Sodium: 600mg
- Fiber: 0g

HEALTHY CAULIFLOWER HASH BROWNS

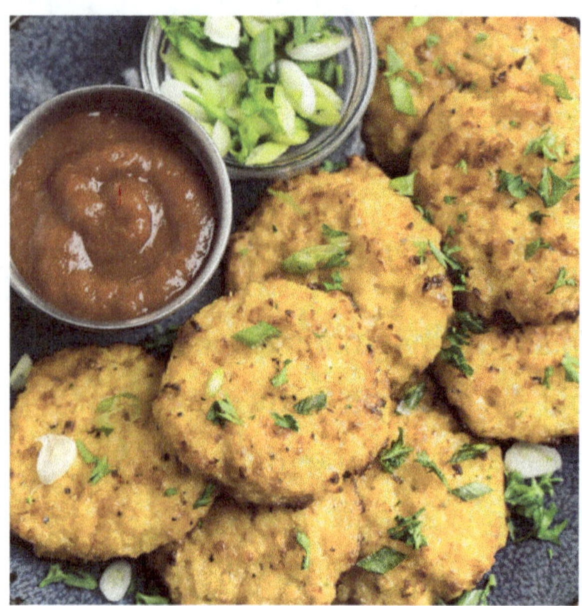

Cook Time: 40 Mins

Serving Size: 2

INGREDIENTS

- 1 medium head of cauliflower (about 4 cups grated)
- 1 large egg, beaten
- 1/2 cup almond flour
- 1/4 cup finely chopped onion
- 1 garlic clove, minced
- 1/4 cup chopped fresh parsley
- 1/2 teaspoon turmeric powder
- 1/2 teaspoon ground cumin
- 1/4 teaspoon ground black pepper
- 1/4 teaspoon sea salt
- 2 tablespoons olive oil or avocado oil (for frying)

INSTRUCTIONS

- Prepare Cauliflower: Grate the cauliflower, then squeeze out excess moisture using a kitchen towel.
- Mix Ingredients: In a bowl, combine cauliflower, egg, almond flour, onion, garlic, parsley, turmeric, cumin, black pepper, and salt.
- Form Patties: Shape the mixture into 8 patties.
- Cook Hash Browns: Heat 1 tablespoon of oil in a skillet over medium heat. Cook patties for 4-5 minutes on each side until golden brown, adding more oil as needed.

NUTRITIONAL FACTS

- Calories: 120
- Total Fat: 8g
- Cholesterol: 35mg
- Sodium: 180mg
- Total Carbohydrates: 8g
- Protein: 5g

TURKEY MEATBALLS

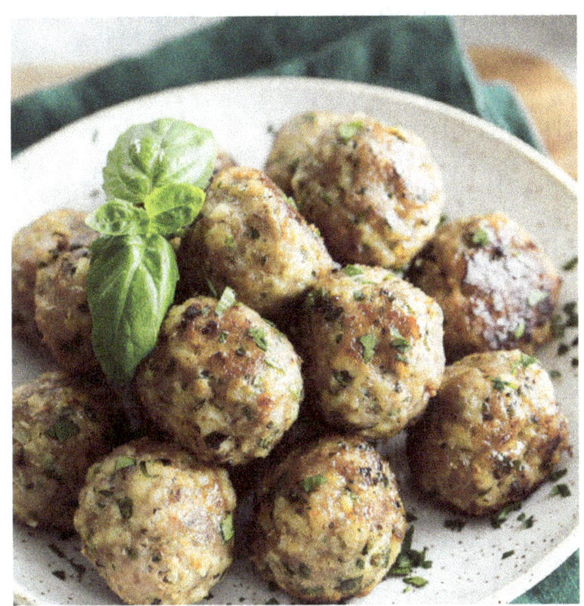

Cook Time: 25 Mins

Serving Size: 4

INGREDIENTS

- 1 lb ground turkey (preferably organic and pasture-raised)
- 1/2 cup finely chopped onion
- 2 cloves garlic, minced
- 1/4 cup finely chopped fresh parsley
- 1/4 cup ground flaxseed
- 1 large egg
- 1 tsp turmeric powder
- 1 tsp ground cumin
- 1/2 tsp ground black pepper
- 1/2 tsp sea salt
- 1 tbsp extra virgin olive oil (for cooking)

INSTRUCTIONS

- Preheat your oven to 375°F (190°C).
- In a large mixing bowl, combine the ground turkey, chopped onion, minced garlic, fresh parsley, ground flaxseed, egg, turmeric powder, ground cumin, ground black pepper, and sea salt.
- Mix all the ingredients thoroughly until well combined.
- Using your hands or a small scoop, shape the mixture into meatballs about 1 1/2 inches in diameter.
- Place the meatballs on a plate or baking sheet lined with parchment paper.
- Heat the extra virgin olive oil in a large skillet over medium-high heat.
- Add the meatballs to the skillet, ensuring they do not touch. You may need to do this in batches.
- Sear the meatballs for about 2-3 minutes on each side, until they are browned all over.

NUTRITIONAL FACTS

- Calories: 180kcal
- Protein: 20g
- Carbohydrates: 5g
- Dietary Fiber: 2g
- Sugars: 1g
- Fat: 8g

INSTRUCTIONS

- Transfer the seared meatballs to a baking dish or a baking sheet lined with parchment paper.
- Place the baking dish or sheet in the preheated oven.
- Bake for 15-20 minutes, or until the meatballs are cooked through and reach an internal temperature of 165°F (74°C).
- Remove the meatballs from the oven and let them rest for a few minutes before serving.

LEMON-BLUEBERRY POKE CAKE

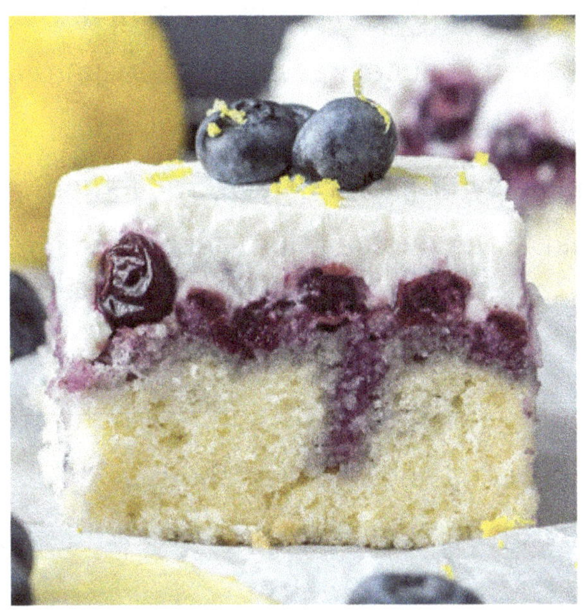

Cook Time: 30 Mins

Serving Size: 9

INGREDIENTS

For the Cake:

- 1 ½ cups almond flour
- ½ cup coconut flour
- 1 teaspoon baking soda
- ½ teaspoon sea salt
- ½ cup unsweetened applesauce
- ½ cup coconut oil, melted
- ½ cup honey or maple syrup
- 3 large eggs
- 1 tablespoon lemon zest (from about 1 lemon)
- 2 tablespoons fresh lemon juice
- 1 teaspoon vanilla extract

For the Blueberry Sauce:

- 2 cups fresh or frozen blueberries
- ¼ cup honey or maple syrup
- 1 tablespoon fresh lemon juice

INSTRUCTIONS

- Preheat your oven to 350°F (175°C). Grease a 9x9-inch baking pan with coconut oil or line it with parchment paper.
- In a medium bowl, whisk together the almond flour, coconut flour, baking soda, and sea salt.
- In a large bowl, mix the applesauce, melted coconut oil, honey (or maple syrup), eggs, lemon zest, lemon juice, and vanilla extract until well combined.
- Gradually add the dry ingredients to the wet ingredients, stirring until just combined. Pour the batter into the prepared baking pan and spread it evenly. Bake for 25-30 minutes, or until a toothpick inserted into the center comes out clean. Allow the cake to cool completely in the pan on a wire rack.

INGREDIENTS

- 1 teaspoon lemon zest
- 1 tablespoon chia seeds (optional, for thickening)

For the Lemon Glaze:

- 1 cup powdered erythritol (or another powdered sugar substitute)
- 2-3 tablespoons fresh lemon juice

NUTRITIONAL FACTS

- Calories: 260kcal
- Total Fat: 15g
- Total Carbohydrates: 28g
- Dietary Fiber: 4g
- Sugars: 18g
- Protein: 5g

INSTRUCTIONS

- While the cake is baking, prepare the blueberry sauce. In a small saucepan, combine the blueberries, honey (or maple syrup), lemon juice, and lemon zest. Cook over medium heat, stirring occasionally, until the blueberries break down and the mixture thickens, about 10 minutes. If using, stir in the chia seeds and cook for another minute. Remove from heat and let cool.
- Once the cake has cooled, use the end of a wooden spoon or a straw to poke holes all over the cake. Pour the cooled blueberry sauce over the cake, spreading it evenly so it seeps into the holes.
- In a small bowl, whisk together the powdered erythritol and lemon juice until smooth. Drizzle the glaze over the top of the cake.
- Refrigerate the cake for at least 1 hour before serving to allow the flavors to meld. Slice and serve chilled.

OATMEAL COOKIE FRUIT PIZZA

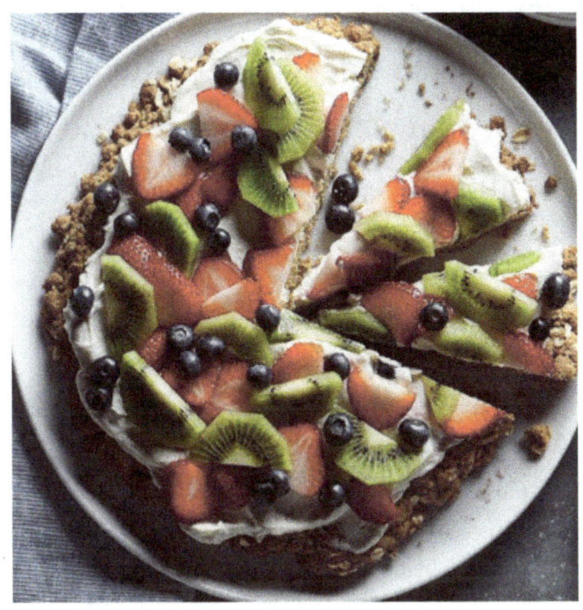

Cook Time: 20 Mins

Serving Size: 8

INGREDIENTS

- For the oatmeal cookie crust:
- 1 1/2 cups rolled oats
- 1/2 cup almond flour
- 1/4 cup coconut oil, melted
- 1/4 cup pure maple syrup
- 1 teaspoon vanilla extract
- 1/2 teaspoon ground cinnamon
- 1/4 teaspoon sea salt
- For the topping:
- 1 cup Greek yogurt (dairy-free yogurt for vegan option)
- 1 teaspoon honey or maple syrup (optional, adjust to taste)
- Assorted fresh fruits such as strawberries, blueberries, kiwi, and oranges, sliced

INSTRUCTIONS

- Preheat your oven to 350°F (175°C). Line a baking sheet with parchment paper.
- In a large bowl, combine rolled oats, almond flour, melted coconut oil, maple syrup, vanilla extract, cinnamon, and sea salt. Mix until well combined.
- Transfer the oatmeal cookie dough onto the prepared baking sheet. Use your hands to press the dough into a round shape, about 1/4 inch thick.
- Bake the oatmeal cookie crust in the preheated oven for 15-18 minutes, or until the edges are golden brown. Remove from the oven and let it cool completely.
- In a small bowl, mix Greek yogurt with honey or maple syrup if using.
- Once the oatmeal cookie crust has cooled, spread the Greek yogurt mixture evenly over the crust.

NUTRITIONAL FACTS

- Calories: 220kcal
- Total Fat: 11g
- Total Carbohydrates: 24g
- Dietary Fiber: 3g
- Sugars: 10g
- Protein: 7g

INSTRUCTIONS

- Arrange the sliced fruits on top of the yogurt layer in a decorative pattern.
- Slice the fruit pizza into wedges and serve immediately.

PEANUT BUTTER CUPS

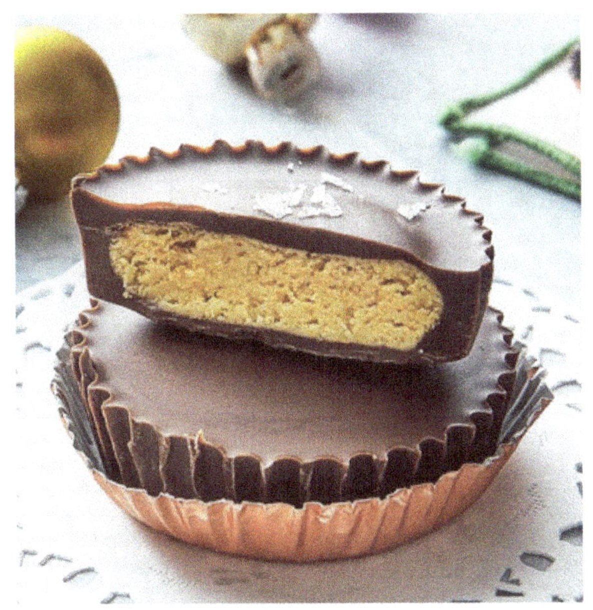

Cook Time: 30 Mins

Serving Size: 4

INGREDIENTS

- 1/2 cup coconut oil
- 1/2 cup unsweetened cocoa powder
- 1/4 cup honey or maple syrup (adjust to taste)
- 1/2 cup natural peanut butter (no added sugar or oils)
- 1 teaspoon vanilla extract
- Pinch of salt (optional)
- Chopped nuts or seeds (optional, for topping)

INSTRUCTIONS

- Melt coconut oil, then whisk in cocoa powder and sweetener.
- Mix peanut butter, vanilla, and salt.
- Line mini muffin tin.
- Layer chocolate mixture, peanut butter, then more chocolate into each liner.
- Optional: top with nuts/seeds.
- Freeze for 30 minutes.
- Store in the refrigerator until serving.

NUTRITIONAL FACTS

- Calories: Approximately 150
- Total Fat: 12g
- Total Carbohydrates: 9g
- Dietary Fiber: 2g
- Sugars: 5g
- Protein: 3g

NOTE:

ALMOND COCONUT MACAROONS

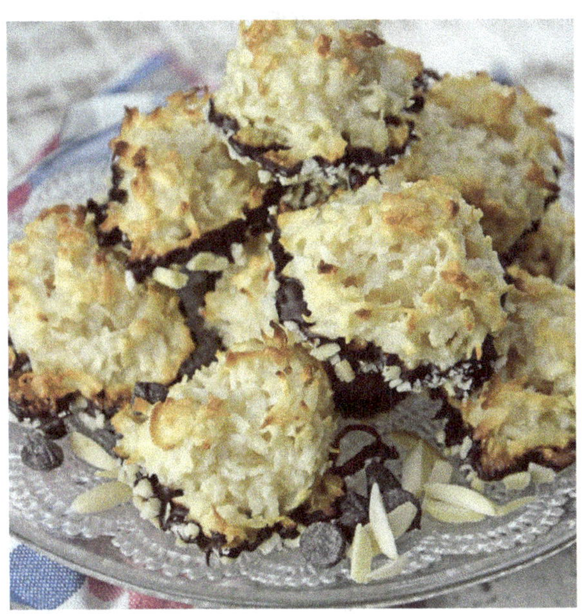

Cook Time: 15 Mins

Serving Size: 20

INGREDIENTS

- 2 cups unsweetened shredded coconut
- 1 cup almond flour
- 1/2 cup honey or maple syrup (for sweetness, optional)
- 1/4 cup coconut oil, melted
- 2 teaspoons vanilla extract
- 1/4 teaspoon sea salt
- 2 tablespoons almond milk (if needed for consistency)
- Optional: 1/4 cup chopped almonds or almond slices for topping

INSTRUCTIONS

- Preheat your oven to 350°F (175°C). Line a baking sheet with parchment paper.
- In a large bowl, mix together the shredded coconut, almond flour, honey or maple syrup (if using), melted coconut oil, vanilla extract, and sea salt until well combined.
- If the mixture seems too dry, add almond milk gradually until it reaches a moist but moldable consistency.
- Using a cookie scoop or your hands, form the mixture into small balls and place them on the prepared baking sheet. If desired, press a few chopped almonds or almond slices onto the top of each macaroon for added crunch.
- Bake in the preheated oven for 12-15 minutes, or until the macaroons are lightly golden brown around the edges.

NUTRITIONAL FACTS

- Calories: 120 kcal
- Total Fat: 10g
- Saturated Fat: 8g
- Sodium: 35mg
- Total Carbohydrates: 7g
- Dietary Fiber: 2g
- Sugars: 4g
- Protein: 1.5g

INSTRUCTIONS

- Remove from the oven and let the macaroons cool on the baking sheet for 5 minutes before transferring them to a wire rack to cool completely.

CHERRY ALMOND CLAFOUTIS

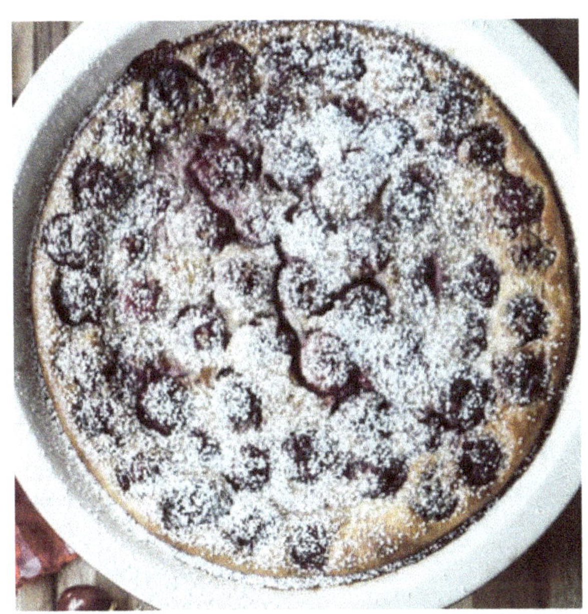

Cook Time: 40 Mins

Serving Size: 6

INGREDIENTS

- 2 cups fresh cherries, pitted
- 1/2 cup almond flour
- 1/4 cup honey or maple syrup
- 3 large eggs
- 1 cup unsweetened almond milk
- 1 teaspoon vanilla extract
- 1/4 teaspoon almond extract
- Pinch of salt
- Sliced almonds for garnish (optional)

NUTRITIONAL FACTS

- Calories: 180kcal | Total Fat: 8g
- Total Carbohydrates: 23g
- Dietary Fiber: 2g
- Sugars: 18g
- Protein: 5g

INSTRUCTIONS

- Preheat your oven to 350°F (175°C). Grease a 9-inch pie dish or baking dish with coconut oil or non-stick cooking spray.
- Arrange the pitted cherries evenly in the bottom of the dish.
- In a mixing bowl, whisk together almond flour, honey or maple syrup, eggs, almond milk, vanilla extract, almond extract, and salt until smooth.
- Pour the batter over the cherries in the dish.
- Optional: Sprinkle sliced almonds over the top of the batter for added crunch.
- Bake in the preheated oven for 35-40 minutes, or until the clafoutis is set and golden brown on top.
- Remove from the oven and let it cool for a few minutes before serving.
- Serve warm or at room temperature. Enjoy!

NOTE:

SPICED BAKED APPLES

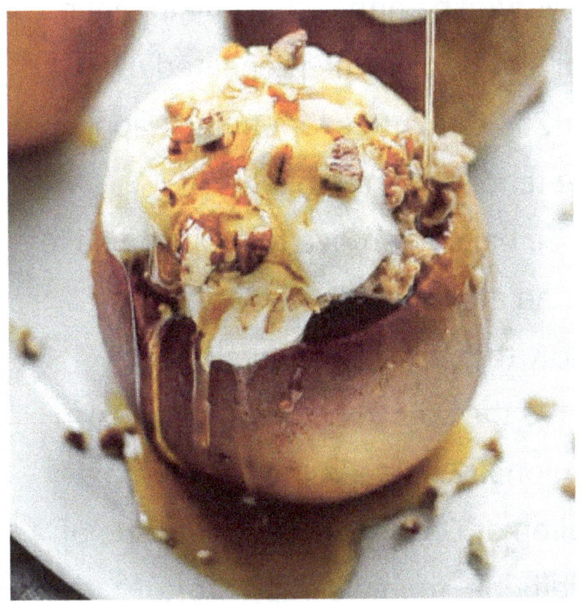

Cook Time: 40 Mins

Serving Size: 4

INGREDIENTS

- 4 large apples (such as Granny Smith or Honeycrisp)
- 2 tablespoons maple syrup or honey
- 1 tablespoon melted coconut oil or olive oil
- 1 teaspoon ground cinnamon
- 1/2 teaspoon ground ginger
- 1/4 teaspoon ground nutmeg
- 1/4 teaspoon ground cloves
- 1/4 cup chopped walnuts or pecans (optional)
- Fresh lemon juice (from 1 lemon)
- Pinch of salt

INSTRUCTIONS

- Preheat your oven to 375°F (190°C).
- Core the apples: Using an apple corer or a sharp knife, carefully remove the cores from the apples without cutting all the way through the bottom. You want to create a well in the center for the filling.
- In a small bowl, mix together the maple syrup or honey, melted coconut oil or olive oil, ground cinnamon, ground ginger, ground nutmeg, ground cloves, chopped nuts (if using), fresh lemon juice, and a pinch of salt.
- Place the cored apples in a baking dish, standing upright. If they're wobbly, you can slice a small piece off the bottom to create a stable base.
- Fill each apple with the spiced mixture, dividing it evenly among them. You can use a spoon to press the filling down into the apples if needed.

NUTRITIONAL FACTS

- Calories: 180kcal
- Total Fat: 7g
- Total Carbohydrates: 31g
- Dietary Fiber: 5g
- Sugars: 22g
- Protein: 1g

INSTRUCTIONS

- Cover the baking dish with aluminum foil and bake in the preheated oven for 25-30 minutes, or until the apples are tender but not mushy.
- Once baked, remove the foil and bake for an additional 5-10 minutes to allow the tops to brown slightly.
- Serve the spiced baked apples warm. Optionally, you can top them with a dollop of Greek yogurt or a drizzle of additional maple syrup before serving.

CINNAMON ROASTED ALMONDS

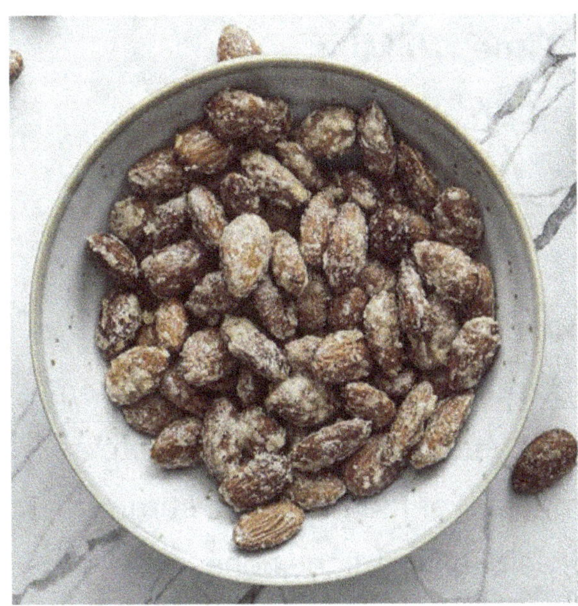

Cook Time: 25 Mins

Serving Size: 1/4 cup

INGREDIENTS

- 2 cups raw almonds
- 1 tablespoon coconut oil (melted)
- 2 tablespoons maple syrup or honey
- 1 teaspoon ground cinnamon
- 1/4 teaspoon sea salt

NUTRITIONAL FACTS

- Calories: 200kcal
- Total Fat: 17g
- Saturated Fat: 2g
- Cholesterol: 0mg
- Sodium: 60mg
- Total Carbohydrates: 8g
- Dietary Fiber: 4g
- Sugars: 3g
- Protein: 7g

INSTRUCTIONS

- Preheat your oven to 300°F (150°C).
- In a bowl, mix together the melted coconut oil, maple syrup (or honey), ground cinnamon, and sea salt.
- Add the raw almonds to the bowl and toss until they are evenly coated with the mixture.
- Spread the almonds out in a single layer on a baking sheet lined with parchment paper.
- Roast the almonds in the preheated oven for about 20-25 minutes, stirring occasionally, until they are golden brown and fragrant.
- Remove the almonds from the oven and let them cool completely before serving.
- Once cooled, store the cinnamon roasted almonds in an airtight container.

GINGER PEAR SORBET

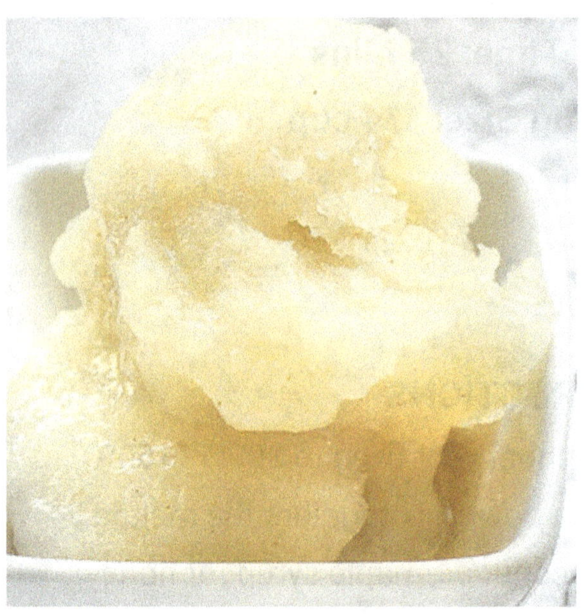

Cook Time: 10 Mins

Serving Size: 4

INGREDIENTS

- 4 ripe pears, peeled, cored, and chopped
- 1 tablespoon freshly grated ginger
- 1/4 cup honey (adjust to taste)
- 1/4 cup water
- 1 tablespoon lemon juice

NUTRITIONAL FACTS

- Calories: 120
- Total Fat: 0g
- Saturated Fat: 0g
- Cholesterol: 0mg
- Sodium: 1mg
- Total Carbohydrate: 32g
- Dietary Fiber: 4g
- Sugars: 24g
- Protein: 1g

INSTRUCTIONS

- In a small saucepan, combine water, honey, and grated ginger. Bring to a simmer over medium heat, stirring occasionally until the honey is dissolved. Remove from heat and let it cool completely.
- In a blender or food processor, blend the chopped pears and lemon juice until smooth.
- Add the cooled ginger-honey syrup to the pear mixture and blend until well combined.
- Pour the mixture into an ice cream maker and churn according to the manufacturer's instructions until it reaches a sorbet consistency.
- Transfer the sorbet to a freezer-safe container and freeze for at least 2 hours or until firm.
- Before serving, let the sorbet sit at room temperature for a few minutes to soften slightly. Scoop into bowls or cones and enjoy!

TURMERIC CHAI PUMPKIN MUFFINS

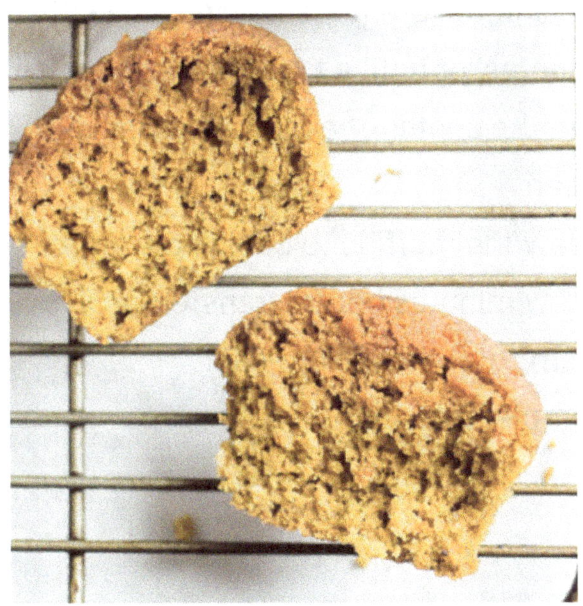

cook Time: 20 Mins

Serving Size: 12 Muffins

INGREDIENTS

- 1 ½ cups whole wheat flour
- 1 cup pumpkin puree
- ½ cup maple syrup or honey
- ⅓ cup coconut oil, melted
- 2 eggs
- 1 teaspoon vanilla extract
- 1 teaspoon ground turmeric
- 1 teaspoon ground cinnamon
- ½ teaspoon ground ginger
- ¼ teaspoon ground cardamom
- ¼ teaspoon ground cloves
- 1 teaspoon baking powder
- ½ teaspoon baking soda
- Pinch of salt
- ½ cup chopped walnuts or pecans (optional)

INSTRUCTIONS

- Preheat your oven to 350°F (175°C). Grease a muffin tin or line it with muffin liners.
- In a large mixing bowl, whisk together the pumpkin puree, maple syrup or honey, melted coconut oil, eggs, and vanilla extract until well combined.
- In a separate bowl, sift together the whole wheat flour, turmeric, cinnamon, ginger, cardamom, cloves, baking powder, baking soda, and salt.
- Gradually add the dry ingredients to the wet ingredients, stirring until just combined. Be careful not to overmix.
- If using, fold in the chopped walnuts or pecans.
- Divide the batter evenly among the prepared muffin cups, filling each about ¾ full.

NUTRITIONAL FACTS

- Calories: 180kcal
- Total Fat: 8g
- Total Carbohydrates: 25g
- Dietary Fiber: 2g
- Sugars: 11g
- Protein: 3g

INSTRUCTIONS

- Bake in the preheated oven for 18-20 minutes, or until a toothpick inserted into the center of a muffin comes out clean.
- Allow the muffins to cool in the tin for a few minutes before transferring them to a wire rack to cool completely.

BEET SUMAC HUMMUS

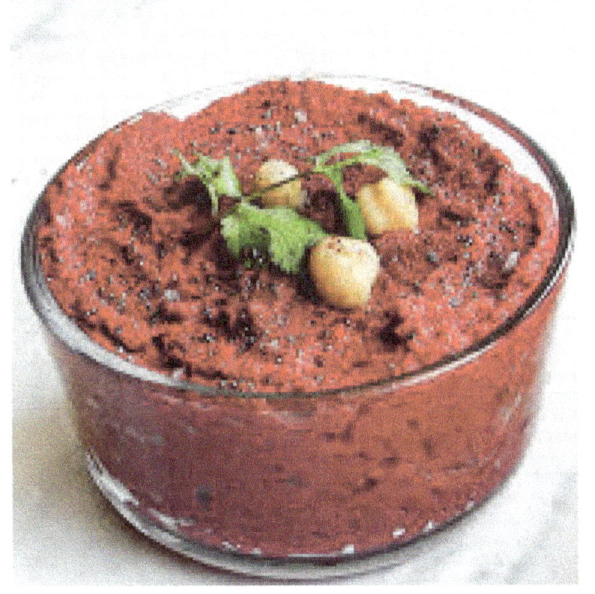

Cook Time: 1 Hour

Serving Size: 8

INGREDIENTS

- 1 can (15 ounces) chickpeas, drained and rinsed
- 2 medium beets, roasted and peeled
- 2 cloves garlic, minced
- 3 tablespoons tahini
- 3 tablespoons lemon juice
- 1 teaspoon ground sumac
- 2 tablespoons extra virgin olive oil
- Salt to taste
- Water (as needed for desired consistency)

NUTRITIONAL FACTS

- Calories: 120kcal | Total Fat: 7g
- Carbohydrates: 12g | Fiber: 3g
- Sugars: 2g | Protein: 4g

INSTRUCTIONS

- Preheat the oven to 400°F (200°C). Wrap each beet individually in aluminum foil and place on a baking sheet. Roast for about 45-60 minutes, or until the beets are tender when pierced with a fork. Let them cool, then peel and dice the beets.

- In a food processor, combine the chickpeas, roasted beets, minced garlic, tahini, lemon juice, and ground sumac. Process until smooth.

- While the food processor is running, drizzle in the olive oil. If the hummus is too thick, add water, a tablespoon at a time, until you reach your desired consistency.

- Add salt to taste and adjust other seasonings if necessary. Process again to incorporate.

- Transfer the hummus to a serving dish. Drizzle with a little extra olive oil and sprinkle with sumac for garnish if desired.

NOTE:

10-MINUTE SPICY TUNA ROLLS

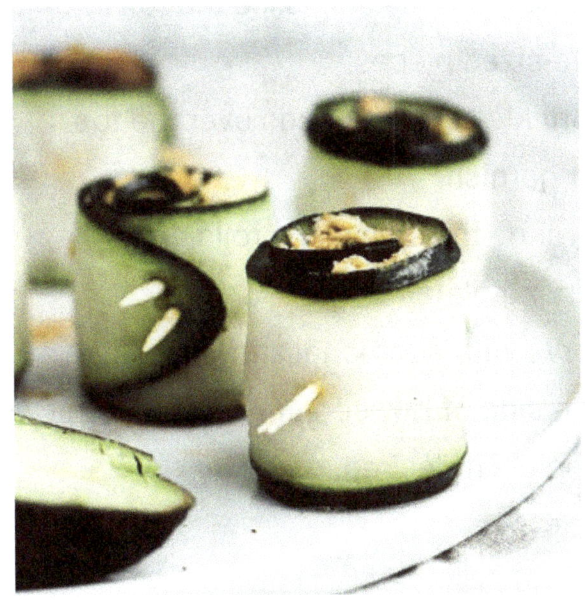

Prep Time: 10 Mins

Serving Size: 4

INGREDIENTS

For the Tuna Filling:

- 1 can (5 oz) of tuna packed in water, drained
- 1 tablespoon plain Greek yogurt (unsweetened, low-fat)
- 1 teaspoon sriracha sauce (adjust to taste)
- 1 teaspoon sesame oil
- 1 teaspoon finely chopped green onions
- 1 teaspoon finely chopped cilantro (optional)
- 1/2 teaspoon freshly grated ginger
- 1/2 teaspoon turmeric powder

INSTRUCTIONS

- In a medium bowl, combine the drained tuna, Greek yogurt, sriracha sauce, sesame oil, green onions, cilantro (if using), grated ginger, and turmeric powder.
- Mix well until all ingredients are evenly combined.
- Lay a nori sheet on a flat surface, shiny side down.
- Place a thin layer of cucumber strips on the nori sheet, leaving about an inch at the top edge of the nori.
- Spread a layer of the spicy tuna mixture over the cucumber strips.
- Place a few avocado slices on top of the tuna mixture.
- Starting from the bottom edge, roll the nori tightly over the filling, pressing firmly to ensure it sticks together.
- Use a little water to seal the edge of the nori sheet.

INGREDIENTS

For the Rolls:

- 1 large cucumber, cut into thin strips (for an anti-inflammatory option instead of rice)
- 1 avocado, thinly sliced
- 4 nori sheets
- Sesame seeds for garnish

NUTRITIONAL FACTS

- Calories: 200kcal
- Protein: 15g
- Fat: 12g
- Saturated Fat: 2g
- Carbohydrates: 8g
- Fiber: 4g
- Sugars: 2g

INSTRUCTIONS

- Using a sharp knife, slice the roll into bite-sized pieces.
- Sprinkle sesame seeds over the top for garnish.
- Arrange the spicy tuna rolls on a serving plate.
- Serve with additional sriracha sauce or a side of low-sodium soy sauce for dipping, if desired.

NOTE:

NOTE:

NOTE:

NOTE:

NOTE:

NOTE:

NOTE:

NOTE:

NOTE:

NOTE: